IT TAKES LOTS
OF COURAGE AND
LOVING HEART,
TO BE A NURSE

It Takes Lots of Courage and Loving Heart, To Be A Nurse

Kehinde Ikuomenisan, RN, MSN

To order additional copies of this book, contact:
Xlibris Corporation
1-888-795-4274
www.Xlibris.com
Orders@Xlibris.com
68572

CONTENTS

This book is a letter to my friends who had expressed interest in majoring in nursing at the local college where they lived. Most of them had graduated from college in a different field, and had been struggling for years to find employment in their respective chosen disciplines.

INTRODUCTION

This book was a letter to my friends who had expressed interest in majoring in nursing at the local college where they lived. Most of them had graduated from college in a different field, and had been struggling for years to find employment in their respective chosen disciplines.

The book detailed my experiences and experiences of my nursing colleagues both during our college days and after graduation from college. It would have been easier to tell my friends to enter the nursing profession because of the shortages and because it offers fruitful employment, but I chose to let them decide for themselves. Nursing school was not easy. The program was difficult and more strenuous than that of medical school. The program instructors were like werewolves. They were not easy to please. The nursing students were treated with disrespect and indignity. The assignments were extremely difficult. The method of teaching and learning were different from that of high school. A student has to be exceptionally careful, humble, and determined to be all he or she could be to graduate.

After graduation, there were other difficulties such as intimidations, abuse, and threats from colleagues, patients, their families, friends, and other disciplines. However, as a nurse, there are un-comparable rewards that we often enjoy such as the thank you that we receive from patients, and the smiles and the joy of savings stranger's life.

I am a nurse and I am proud to be a nurse. I would not trade it for any other profession. I wanted my friends to see the world of nursing through the eyes of a nurse and make up their mind to see if they are nursing materials.

Dear friend,

I understand that you are inquiring about the school of nursing because you have genuine interest in becoming a nurse. It is a good profession, but it has its problems just like any other profession. I am not going to recommend that you make this profession your own, but I would let you decide on your own as to whether you should be a nurse or not. The following are some nursing experiences which I selectively chose to share with you. It is not to scare you, but to enable to get a deeper understanding of the profession today, and where it may be heading in the near future.

Nursing profession evolved as a selfless, humane, empathetic, and caring profession. It was a not a favorable profession among the children or relatives of the wealthy, affluent or the most famous. Caring for people is a hard and stressful occupation. The wealthy and the affluent do not have any affinity for such occupation, and would not want to see their children or relative performing such occupation.

Ask any children of the rich who was responsible for their upbringing, they would tell you it was not their mother and father. It was either the maid or the nanny or some poor hired help who change their diapers, fed them, responded to their needs and taught them most of the basic foundation of early childhood. Every house from the averagely rich to the multimillion dollar jackasses in America, Europe, Asia, and Africa has a maid or hired help to care for the children and oversee house chores. The rich women and men are never at home. They are either at work, on business trips, or shopping somewhere. All the complications and the stress that comes with nursing children and providing care for the sick at the home of the wealthy are done by children of the poor or some other hired hands, even today.

As a matter of fact, the early nurses, besides Nightingale, were nuns and children of the poor. This was supported by historical development of nursing as recorded in one of the fundamental of nursing books. With the Reformation, there was a decline in people's interest in and support of the church and religion. This change in people's interest to support the work of the church resulted in an era in nursing history known as the "dark period." The hospitals were unsanitary places, and the work was overwhelming in comparison to what we see in health care today. Nursing care was provided by women who were frequently described as drunk, heartless, and immoral. They were expected to carry out the housework of the hospital, such as wash the laundry, and do all the cleaning for very little reward. They were not respected, and were considered the dregs of the society. They were not considered suitable marriage mates by many in the society because of their profession, and also because of the myths of their chosen profession. The nurses were regarded as doctor's assistant and were believed to often have illicit affairs with the doctors in the wards, and sometimes with patients. These myths, I believed, gave rise to the other myths that nurses were prostitutes, and also need not be trusted. Many people call them whores or prostitutes, silently. The myths were results of society's ignorance and laziness. The word should have been illiteracy rather than ignorance, because there are many secularly educated people in the world that are still illiterate relative to nursing profession.

The men in nursing are viewed by many in the society as weird or homosexual. This is because those people see the profession as only for female. They had forgotten or they did not know or never read that soldiers in the military, a profession previously designated only for men, had some men as nurses. They were chosen few who nursed their comrade wounds and empathizes with those who lost loved ones at war. These men were at times commanded to do what they do by their captain, sergeant, or other designated commander at their posts, but many willingly out of courage, loving heart, and empathy submitted to help their fellow soldiers as nurses. There were others who were not soldiers, but were deputized as nurses too during crises. They were fathers, brothers, uncles, cousins, and friends of people in need of help and out of compassion, willingly gave themselves as nurses for that particular moment. For example, during a crisis in which about one thousand people were presumed dead under a collapsed three stories building, men were the first to rush to the aide of those who were alive, and initiate the start of searching for the dead and the living. If you watch the television, which does not provide good news, but tragedy, you will see that in all the televised events, men are in the forefront of providing care as nurses or assistant to some medical personnel. If you are a man, do not listen to the myths that men in nursing are homosexual, because it is not true, however, if you chose this as a profession, and you are a male, you will encounter patients or relatives who will think of you as homosexual or weird.

As a man in nursing, some will not see you as a nurse, even when your identification identifies you as a registered nurse. They would first thought of you as an orderly, a male nursing assistant. You may correct them, but they would still not believe. You would be thrown all over the place as a result of your gender. Everyone will require that you assist them in lifting patients, moving furniture, beds, transferring patients, and everything else requiring human powers. All these you have to do in addition to your given assignment. Unfortunately, you are not allowed to decline to assist those nursing assistant, patients, or other nurses. If you declined, you will be reported, and if an incident occurred as a result of your failure to assist, you could be disciplined or suspended or even terminated. You are the man not only on your unit, but for other ward or unit too. They would call you or demand that you come to help them and when you need help, they will tell you that they are busy or have backache or shoulder pain. You work three times as hard as the female nurses, but you get paid the same. Your patients would be selected for you, out of the rejected ones by the female nurses. This means that you will have the most difficult patients.

Nursing have struggled to be recognized as a profession, and not as a doctor assistant or a prostitute or inhumane and apathetic, but as an entity devoted to providing safe, effective, empathetic, holistic, and culturally competent care in collaborations with other health care profession for the best outcomes for every patient, client, or resident, depending on the nursing spectrum a nurse belong. To develop a curriculum for nursing, to address issues that are pertinent to nursing care, which are the care of the social, physical, psychological, emotional, and spiritual needs of the patient and his or her family. Nursing had to borrow from other disciplines. Some appropriate knowledge was taken from sociology, chemistry, biology, physics, psychology, health sciences, anatomy and physiology, and religion to create effective foundation of nursing. These efforts were to prepare nurses for effective care of their patients and family. Nursing school were developed to provide necessary education that would equipped nurses to provide adequate and effective nursing care relative to the changing global health care demands.

Nursing school admission is not the same as the medical school admissions; however, there are some similarities. For example, prior to being accepted into the nursing program, the applicants must complete some appropriate classes such as chemistry, anatomy and physiology, psychology, sociology, English, and mathematics. The applicant's grade in those classes determines whether they will be immediately accepted into the nursing program or they have to retake the classes for a grade of "B" or better. Each college of nursing is different, but the method of admission is the same.

Once in the program, you are not guaranteed graduation or completion of the program. Your goal or dream of becoming a nurse, wholly rest in the hands of the lecturers, and the nursing program coordinator. They determine whether you move on to the next phase or are left behind or drop out of the nursing program. You may influence the outcomes of their decisions in some ways, and this depends on how bad you really want to be a nurse. In most cases, they control everything regarding who proceed or who get left behind or thrown out. This is how we evolve in a metamorphic process, in the profession called nursing. The educational environment were created to prepare us for the uncomfortable real world of health care, which changes daily due to lack of trust, diverse cultural health beliefs, illiteracy and ignorance of the nursing profession.

We all decided to become nurses for different reasons, but majority of us chose this profession for answers to some unanswered questions, and for the love of people, especially the ill patients. We wanted to touch the lives of people in a way their family are unable to, and thereby put a smile on their faces.

The first phase of the nursing education involved the curiosity of the nursing program coordinators, as to why we wanted to be nurses. We were told to write a paragraph of why we chose this as a profession. There were numerous and factual reasons many applied to the schools of nursing, as our responses were read back to us. One student had lost many brothers and sisters in death, while she was young. She could not understand, but hope by becoming a nurse, she would find answers and prevent the same from happening in her family in the future. She was hoping to save other people's lives, but also her own. Another student hope by becoming a nurse, she could give back, as a reward for the help she received from a nurse when she was a teenager. At 14 years of age, she was diagnosed with ovarian cancer, and was terrified of the unknown outcome of her illness. In spite of all her anxiety, and anger towards everyone, the only profession empathetic to her suffering during her illness was a nurse. The nurses understood that her anger was a reaction to her diagnosis of cancer, and fear of death from the illness. She received daily support, love, encouragement, instruction, both scripturally, and medically from the nurses. It was the support from the nurses, which motivated her to accept treatment for her cancer and thereby saved her life.

Other students claimed they wanted to be a nurse to make money, to be able to pay their daily expenses, and lived comfortably. Nothing is wrong with money as a reason for choosing a profession. To be good in that profession, one must loved it or have other reasons besides money. If the money part is inadequate, the love of the profession should provide the motivation to stay in the profession. It was just like my father once said about factors which helps a person stayed with the same employment until retirement. "There are three reasons a person stays on the job until retirement, the love of the profession, the friends they have made, and the treatment of their employer. Love of the profession reduces the stress and helps you to deal with encountered problems daily. Friends are there to provide support in any form to urge you on and to help you deal with personal problems on the job. The treatment of the employer includes the benefits and salary provided by the employer in comparison to other employer in the same business. Money should not be a priority for getting into the nursing profession. Putting the love of money above the love or care of the ill, could crowd a person's judgment, and prevent the person from doing the honorable thing. After all, the same eventuality befalls everyone. Just as the poor are dying, so the rich too, are dying. It has never happened or written or proven that money saved a wealthy person from death. It may buy you some time when you are ill through expensive innovative health care, sometimes, but not forever.

With that baring of souls, the educational experiences began. Every day, before the nursing lectures, we had quizzes regarding the nursing topic for the day. The quizzes were not easy, and were tricky. You had to have read between the lines and memorized the ten to twenty long chapters of the nursing textbooks to get everything correct on the quizzes. We all tried. We studied and studied. When things did not work the way we planned, some of us bought more books on the topics to gather more information. Every semester, we all spent more money on books. We bought the required and the recommended textbooks, and any other nursing books we believed or we were told would help in preparing us for the class quizzes, in getting better grades and better at clinical aspect of each class of the nursing profession.

It was very stressful for many of us, because it was our first college experience, and things were done differently. We were expecting to be spoon-fed or to get every lecture or topic or course dissected for our understanding. We were not expecting to have to do much reading, memorizing, and meditating on what we read for our ultimate understanding. We were adult learners, but we expect our teacher to teach us rather than leave the responsibility of teaching and learning to us. All we were expecting after every class was to review the information provided by our instructors or professors, and would be acing all the quizzes and the exams. This was not what happened. We got a summary of the topic, and were left to read, understand, and make our own notes.

The pedagogy theory of learning was what we were expecting. It was extremely useful and practical for our learning when we were little. We did not expect things to have changed. We still expect the teacher to teach. After all, that is what teachers were supposed to do. Our principle was that if a student is failing or failed, it is the fault of the teacher. We all were of the opinion that teachers must ensure that student learn by regularly evaluating teaching tools, and other systems of learning. We eventually realize that the evaluations of teaching and learning were done regularly through quizzes and exams. The only problem was, andragogy was the theory of learning employed by our instructors and professors. Dr. Malcolm S. Knowles (1970) developed the adult learning theory for adult learners; and is being used by teachers to help adult learn. It makes learning the responsibility of the adult learners, and not the responsibility of the teacher.

Now, we found ourselves in a different learning environment, which made it seems we were at war. In a way, we were at war. A different kind of war for trust, freedom, respect, information, understanding of everything within the nursing educational environment, to be all we could be in the world of nursing. The war began with the quizzes, the exams and the high demands of the nursing programs and the struggles to prove ourselves to the nursing instructors, professors, clinicians, and the nursing department, that we were nursing materials.

The nursing coordinator and the instructors began to use scare tactics as a motivational tool for us to do better on the quizzes and the exams. They were ignorant of today's students of nursing, and were of the opinion that we were not studying our nursing books, as we should. Most students of nursing today are not single; neither do they live with their parents. They are either married with children or single with children and other domestic responsibilities. They have to juggle home, work, and educational life. They have to prioritize often, but ensure that all activities balance without any neglect. The coordinators of the nursing programs did not do the needed research because they felt it was not their responsibilities to impart knowledge, rather it was our responsibilities to acquire knowledge.

If I remembered correctly, on many occasions, the nursing coordinator threatened to fail or drop or thrown out many students from the nursing program. We did not think it was possible for her to do so. We assumed that education was a right and not a privilege, and as such, none of us could be thrown out of the program. Then, we began to hear rumors that foreign students or those students whom English was not their first language would be thrown out of the program. The excuse given for that rumor was that, there were research done by some idiots that students whom English is not their first language often fail or never passed the NCLEX-RN the first or the second or the third or the fourth try.

During the first semester, many students were either dropped or decided to transfer to another school, to fulfill their dreams of becoming a nurse. The pressure not to fail or be dropped out of the program now dawn on us. Many students, whom English was not their first language, began to panic and frustrated. It appeared to them that regardless of their earnest efforts in the nursing program, they would be failed. Many decided to take their case to the president and dean of the colleges and the universities. The case was presented to the deans and the presidents of the nursing schools. They acted like they were unaware of what was happening at the college nursing departments. After all they wanted the glory of having 100% state board of nursing success. It was supposed to be the criteria for the National League of Nursing Accreditation. They promised to look into the matter. They never did, and if they did, we never knew the outcome of the discussion regarding scare tactics of the school of nursing.

The following semester we witnessed a huge dropped in the Spanish and African languages speaking students from the nursing program. The class continues to get smaller, and smaller. Those who were affected were the brightest student, except that English was not their first language. Those of us, who were still in the program felt worse for those students, but were too selfish to fight. We did not want to become another casualty of the bad decisions of the nursing faculty. Many students resigned from their jobs, and many began to neglect their domestic life just to keep up with the expectations of the nursing programs. I particularly remembered three students who lost their husbands during the third and fourth semester of the nursing program.

One of the three students who lost their husbands arrived at the clinical site one morning with peri-orbital hematoma. Her husband had beaten her up badly that she did not care to examine the damage before leaving the house. Or it was the anxiety of keeping up with the nursing program or not failing the nursing program that numbed her pain or make it impossible for her to feel any pain from the beaten she took from her husband. She wore dark glasses to conceive the marks of the abuse, but had to remove it for the clinical practicum.

She belongs to that group of foreign women, whose abuses often never get reported to the authority. She came from West Africa to meet her husband. She was happy to be in the United States with the man she loved. She had a dream of going to college, but had to be postponed because her husband did not think it was time. After seven years and six children, she finally got the courage to go to school. It was as if every year she sneezed, and a baby dropped out of her private part. It was difficult to imagine that she gets pregnant after each child every year. Her husband thought she should stay home to care for him and the children. She did not have any bank account or job or pension. She was depended on her husband for everything, but she kept seeing advertisement on the television, which reminded her that her husband may leave some day and she would be left alone to provide for the children.

The anxiety of being alone with nothing financially to provide for her children motivated her to want to arm herself with nursing education with which to work and care for herself and her children. In addition, she needed money to help her brothers, sisters, and parents back in their poor West African country.

She discussed the educational plan with her husband, who was not interested or did not care about her educational plans. He brought her here for companionship and for her to breed like chicken or cow or goat. She was the baby manufacturing plants, and he was the owner or the proprietor of the establishment. This was what she had been doing for the past seven years, breeding. She could not believe that her life would not change in spite of the fact that she was no longer in her village.

Her parent had reluctantly put her through high school. Providing education to a girl was a waste of financial resources, because she would soon leave home to be a wife to someone else. It was the traditional belief and the consensus not to even try to provide female children with secular education. Her mother never attended elementary school. She was told to consider herself very lucky to have had the opportunity of secular education beyond the elementary school education.

She had worked on the farm with her parents until a man arrived to ask for her hand in marriage for his son in the United States of America. She was delighted, and her parents considered it an honor. They did not care who the son of the man was or what her personalities were, they were just thrilled that their daughter would be married, and would be going to America. The girl was excited too, because she saw an opportunity to be the first girl in her family to attend school beyond high school education. She had dreamt of attending a university ever since she read a book published by Cambridge University of England.

Going to America, she thought would afford her the opportunity of advancing her education. The day arrived and all the necessary marriage ceremonies were done. The daughter cautioned her parents not to ask for too much, since she would be going to America to live with her husband. She also emphasized that asking for too much money for dowry may delay the wedding or cause the man to pick somebody else for his son for a wife.

She was right about her assumptions because such was the customs in her village. The girl's parents often ask for huge dowry as if they were auctioning off their daughters. It often seems that way because the man always reminded his wife that he paid a lot of money to acquire her as a property. The family did not ask for any dowry, they even bought gifts for their son-in-law when their daughter was traveling to the airport to board the plane to meet her husband.

Although, her husband did not pay any dowry, he acted like he did. She was to be a housewife. This was not communicated to her by her husband, but the intention was there. She was oriented to the use of everything in the house like a new employee. She was observed in demonstrating the correct and appropriate use of all domestic machines. She received series of kisses, and sexual pleasures from her husband as a certificate of completion and correct demonstration of instructions. At that moment, she became his slave. She had had sex before, but never to the point of orgasm and not in the way she had recently experienced it with her husband in United States. In her mind this was love, and joy she had to make sure no one interfere with. She was a devoted wife. She followed her husband's wishes to every letters of instructions, and did as she was told for seven years.

She had six children, and she began to change physically. Her husband began to come home late, and when she gets close to him, he pushed her away, with an excuse of fatigue from work. She could not understand, until she saw her husband kissing another woman.

She had gone to the market with the children to buy foodstuffs. She did not drive because her husband did not think she was good enough to drive his car. She took the bus to the five miles market place, when she got tired of walking or during the rain or during the snow or cold weather.

That day, she saw her husband car, and she decided to run across the street to see who was inside. She saw her husband in the backseat with another West African woman kissing. She was upset, but she did not make a big deal out of it. After all, her husband was entitled to marry a second wife as their custom permits. She said to herself that it must be the new wife her husband was going to marry. "Maybe this is how they do things in America. My husband is testing the new wife before he bring her to the house," she said.

She began to ask many questions of herself, and she almost forgot that she had brought the children to the market with her. She had walked half a mile away from the market when she suddenly realized that her children were still waiting for her on the corner of the street where she had left them. She ran like a mad woman across the busy street with no notice or care for her safety back to where her children were waiting for her. She got to them before anyone noticed that they were there alone with no adult supervision. They were raised in the African way of obedience. They listen and do as they were told. They did not move from the place their mother left them and did not cry. They even saw their mother walking away from their father's car across the street, but did not try to chase after their mother. She had never told them she loved them, but they knew she loved them. If the people around the market place or those walking by had noticed that the children were alone without any adult supervision, they would have called the police or the National Guard or the Federal Bureau of Investigation or the Central Intelligence Agency or the like. This is the United States of America and not Africa. You cannot leave children unattended or without adult supervision, you will be severely dealt with by the justice department. She hugged her children with tears streaming down her cheeks. She walked them across the street with caution. Her legs were wobbling due to her emotional instability. She felt like her knees would buckle, so, she decided to take the bus home with her children.

She had forgotten to buy the foodstuffs. She called her neighbor for the first time to talk to them. She just opened the window, and called out her name. It was not that she was crazy. She did not know her neighbor's telephone number. Even if she did, she had not comprehended how to use it. Her husband often dialed her parents in the village for her. They do not have telephone, but their uncle who was a merchant at Enugu, in Nigeria had a telephone in her shop. Her parents often travelled to his shop at Enugu every market day to receive a call to learn of the gifts or money that had been sent to them through Western Union or other postal means. The only option she had was to shout the name of her neighbor as the custom was in African Village that she had came from. The woman opened the window to look. She saw this girl calling and waving at her to come. It occurred to her that the girl could be psychotic, but she could also be calling her for some help too. She got out of her house and walked to the girl's house. The girl began to ask her questions about American married customs and how men acquire new wives.

The woman thought she was crazy. The girl realized that the woman probably thought she was crazy. She decided to explain to her why she was asking many questions. The woman felt pity for her. She explained to her that a man could only have one woman for a wife in America, and that what her husband was doing was wrong. She was happy. She was delighted that her husband would not have another woman besides her. She would not want to share any other woman with her man. She decided she would tell her husband what she had found out. She reasoned that it was possible that her husband may not know that he could only have one wife in America. She quickly cleaned and dusted the house. Thanked her neighbor for the enlightenment in American culture. She cooked her husband's favorite dish, Ogbono-soup with crumbled dried fish and shrimp. He was to have the soup with pounded-yam.

He returned home as usual. The wife greeted him at the door. He handed over his briefcase to her, and kissed her. She knelt down on her knees at the door to acknowledge respect and devotion to him. They entered the house. He sat on the sofa, and she removed his shoes and loosened his tie for him. She walked him to the bathroom and run the water for him.

After the shower, she set the table with the meal and humbly called him to the table. She brought water in a bowl for him to wash his hand. She was on her knees with the bowl when he was washing his hand. She did not move from her position until he finished washing his hand. He got up and sat next to him until he finished eating. She cleared the table and cleaned the plate.

The husband got up and walked to the living room. He picked up the television remote control, and began to flip through the channels for something to watch. The wife hurried to the living room to tell him what she had found out.

"Darling, I found out today that in America, by law, you could only have one wife. I am sorry that you would not be able to have that woman I saw you with today. I am truly sorry," the girl said.

The husband looked at her, and shouted in a angry voice, "What did you say." The wife, who was ignorant of what was going on with her husband, repeated what she had just said.

The husband could not believe it, and asked, "What woman are you talking about?"

"The one in the car with you this afternoon. I saw your car when I went to the market today. I crossed the street to see who was in the car, and there you were testing the girl with your tongue in her mouth."

"Yeah, right. I was testing the girl for a new wife to help you with the children and the house chores. It is a shame that I cannot marry two women in America. It would have helped in pursuing that college education you so desire to have."

The girl's affect immediately changed to sadness. She desired to advance her education beyond secondary education, but her husband had made it impossible for seven years. For her to hear her husband alluded to her education like this made her happy and also sad. She was happy that her husband had not forgotten about her ambition, and sad, because her husband would not be able to have a second wife to help her care for her children. She truly believed that her husband was testing the woman she saw in the car with him that morning for a possibility of marrying her as a second wife. She also believed that her husband did not know that he could only have one wife in America.

She did not sleep that night and her husband did nothing to help her with her anxiety. The following morning, after her husband had gone to work, she called her neighbor again. She asked her if there was a way for her husband to have a second wife, so she could go to school. The woman tried to laugh, but she noted that she was really innocent rather than ignorant or stupid.

She told her that it was impossible for the girl's husband to have a second wife by law in any country, especially in America. She told her she would let her found out by herself. She took her and her children to the library. She was surprised to see many books. She asked how she could be at the library every day. The lady helped her got a library card and explained to her the rules about the library use. She asked questions and many books were provided for her edification.

She had places to go with her children every morning. She became educated about the morality, rules, regulations and the business of United States of America. She decided she was going to be a nurse. She also knew that her husband was a cheat, and that he was not testing the woman in her car for her suitability for a second wife.

When she got home, she confronted her husband about what she had learned. The husband forbade her from talking to their neighbors, and visiting the library. She demanded to know why, and her husband slapped her hard across the face that her whole body shifted five feet away from where she was originally standing. This was the first time she was ever slapped on her face by anybody. Her father or mother had never beaten her before. She held her face on her palm for sometime staring at her husband, who by now had sat down ready to play with the television remote control, as usual.

Her right eye became blood shot and the skin around the eye had turned black by the following morning. It was obvious to everyone that saw her that she had had an accident or had been beaten by someone. She stayed at home as her husband commanded. She did not go anywhere nor did she venture out of the house into the yard.

The neighbor observed that she had not seen the girl for few weeks, and she had not called for her through the window, as she normally did. She decided to walk to the girl's house and inquire as to what had happened to her. She knocked on the door several times, and there was no response. The girl had seen her, and was afraid that her husband might be upset if she let the neighbor into the house. She stood still for some time, and when the raps on the door stopped, she went to the door. The lady was just about living. She turned to look at the door again, and she saw the girl standing by the door. She spoke to her and she could tell that something was wrong. She inquired if her husband had abused her, and she replied that she had fallen into the tub while she was bathing the children.

The woman knew she was lying, but she did not know if she should get involved. She asked why she had not seen her for weeks, and the girl began to cry. The woman consoled her and asked how she could help her. She explained to her how women are treated in her village and how she had dreamt of having the best education to help her family back in the village. She wanted to be educated as a woman to enlighten the villagers that women and men should have the privilege of secular education because they are both equal in the eyes of God. The woman agreed, because she was educated too. She had a master degree in sociology. She promised to help the girl get into college and she did. Her husband was not happy. He tolerated her attending classes as long as she could be home in time to cook his food.

This particular day, the nursing student had to prepare for final examination. She called her husband to inform him that she would be getting home late. She explained the situation to him. The husband informed her that she could be late as long as she wanted to, but his food must be ready when he gets home. She called the baby-sitter, who was also was an African. She told her to help prepare some food for her husband because she may be a little late coming home this evening due to the group study she was having at the college. The baby-sitter understood. She was going to the same school too, but majoring in a different career. She prepared the husband favorite food the way her tribe prepares them.

The husband arrived from work. He saw that his wife was not home. He took his bath, and sat down to watch the television. The babysitter left the food on the stove for the husband to serve himself. The husband did not, but waited by the television until his wife returns to serve him.

His wife got home. Greeted him as the customs demanded. She knelt on her knees, and she said "Good evening my husband. How was your day? Have you eaten? I had told the baby-sitter to prepare your favorite food for you. Did she give it to you?"

The husband looked at her, and asked, "Am I married to the baby-sitter now? Eh! You ungrateful bastard, I brought you to this country as a favor to your parent. I made you my wife, and that is not enough for you, eh? You want to go to school, eh?"

She replied, "Yes, I want to go to school to learn a skill or trade for which to get a job. I need to do something. I am grateful that you marry me, however, if you had not married me, I probably eventually have a better life." Before she could complete that sentence, her husband slapped her several times. He ran into the bedroom. He removed one of his belts from his pants and began to beat her with it.

It was hard to tell if it was the belt or his fist, which uprooted her front tooth from her mouth. That morning, when her mates saw her at clinical site, she appeared she was in an automobile accident. It was her courage, and the desire to be more than what she was, and the love she had for people, that strengthened her to be able to come for the clinical orientation that day.

As soon as the instructor saw her, she told her she cannot allow her to participate in clinical rotations that day. The student busted into tears. She did not want to fail or get thrown out of the program. She wanted to make sure that she would not be counted absent for that day, and that she would be given the opportunity to repeat the clinical. She appeared to be in pain. Judging from her appearance, she may have been up all night, and who knows, she probably may not have slept at home. She was the first to show up at clinical that morning. We were told she was there at the clinical site, 5:30 A.M. The time for clinical was 8:00 A.M., and she had gotten there at five in the morning.

The following three days, she failed to show up in class. We decided to call her at home, and the husband told us she had travelled to their country to see her parents. He refused to give us any contact telephone number. We continue to try by calling the available number, hoping that we would get her or someone would give us a telephone number or address where she could be reached. By Sunday of the following week, one of the students had gotten a telephone number for us. It was not a residential telephone, but that of a hospital. The girl had been beaten badly that she had miscarriage. She was bleeding profusely that she had to be hospitalized. According to the nurses, she had attempted to sign herself out to attend classes and the nursing clinical practicum that week. She had to be restraint and sedated for her safety. She returned the following week, but only to be dropped from the program, in spite of everyone's knowledge of her domestic problems.

The other student was also beaten by her husband. She lost her tooth in the process. She got home from the library one afternoon. This was after our group study. We had divided ourselves into study groups to assist one another in understanding, digesting, and absorbing all the necessary materials pertaining to passing the quizzes, tests, and class exams. This was done after school. We often spent three to eight hours in the library and on campus every day to study everything pertaining to nursing subject for that week. This was because our books were huge, and contained more information than necessary; and we felt we must complete the book to be confident to pass the course.

Her husband got home from work, and he was expecting her to set his food on the table, and she was not at home. When she got home, the husband asked her where she was coming from. She answered she was just leaving the library. The husband slapped her so hard that one of her tooth fell out. She was bleeding from the gum, but her husband continued to kick her while she was on the floor. He threw hot water from the tap on her. He opened the door and threw her out of the door.

She called one of her friends to come and pick her up. She was taken to the hospital, but she refused to tell the hospital staff or the police how she got her bruises or how she lost her tooth. It was one of those foreigner cases, which Americans and Europeans could never understand. The husband abused the wife, but the wife accepted it as a way of life. Or she wanted to keep the peace between the two in-laws, and refused to report the abuse. These are the unknown abused African women across the United States, and Europe. The tradition permits, and supported it, regardless of the cause. She was worried that if she reported the matter to the police, and her husband was arrested, her in-laws would blame her, and her parents for it. This would result in a big and even fatal war at home between the two in-laws. The matter was never reported to the police. She never missed any nursing classes, but she never went back to her husband. She stayed with her friend until the end of the nursing program.

Different drama continued to occur daily, and the stress of the program was certainly the cause of all the dramas. We continue to fight for the opportunity to become a nurse to care for the sick and the ill. We were never allowed to see our quizzes, or tests or exams. We were called one by one into the nursing office, where two or three of the nursing professors verbally gave us our result. This often caused fear and anxiety that many of us were not able to eat until we were called and informed of how we did on the tests or the exams. The worst times were often during the final exam. Every department would have posted the exam result of their students, but nursing department always held on to their result until four to five weeks later.

The nursing faculty would sit and discussed each student like hospital cases or research study for review. Each would tell what he or she knows about the students, and what he or she feel about whether the student should be passed or failed or allowed to repeat the class or be thrown out of the program. Each instructor's decision was based on interaction with the students during clinical practicum, class lectures, responses to questions in class, result of class quizzes and tests. The quizzes, tests, and the exams carried less weight in their decision making regarding whether a student progress to the next phase or not. One of the clinical instructors explained to my peers that the weightier factors for passing the students depend on the attitude of the students at clinical, perception of the instructors about the student, his or her potential in understanding the materials, and ability to apply the learning materials.

All of the factors are relevant in evaluating a potential applicant for nursing profession, but the secrecy, the scare tactics, and the threats of failing students on the basis of not having English as a first language was purely racist, and was discouraging to many born nurses. In other to stay the course, many of us resolved to "pass through the program courses once." We all wrote in all our books a daily reminder, "I shall pass through this way, but once." We slept nursing, ate nursing, dreamt nursing, date nursing, and married nursing. We did all that we had to do to prevent being the victim of depressive, racist, and antisocial nursing school coordinators.

Others potential nurses had different educational experience, but there were similarities as to the treatment by instructors. The diploma nursing program was like an apprenticeship program of nursing, in which nurses are utilized to run the hospital, while still learning to be a nurse. There were senior nurses, who acted as preceptors or clinical instructors or in some cases as the lecturer and the clinical instructors. The nurses work long hours, including weekends. They had little freedom, and had to be loyal to the doctors and performed their duties according to the instruction of the instructors. Anything less than what was expected could spell expulsion or suspension from the program.

At the end of the fourth of the five semesters devoted only to the nursing program, including one summer, we were beginning to breathe a sigh of relief. We counted ourselves as the lucky ones. It had been a rough journey, which out of fifty-one students, only about nineteenth of the students made it this far. Yet there was still one semester to go. This did not stop the nursing coordinator from her earlier agenda of graduating only those whom she felt would passed the professional registered nursing licensing examination at the first try. She continued to echo the same threat that she would fail some students or drop them from the program. She still believed that there were some students who were not nursing materials, and should not be in the program. She did not mention names, and she was not going to.

At the beginning of that semester, we were all confidents that the race was now our own to complete, without any obstacles. We all decided to prove ourselves that we were nursing materials or that nursing was our calling. We knew we were permitted and were qualified at that moment to sit for the Practical Nurse Licensing Examination. We all decided to apply to take the examination. The nursing coordinator was furious. She was upset that we all put in applications to sit for the exam. She informed us in a loud foaming at the mouth voice, "This is not a practical nursing program. It is a registered nursing program. You are not going to take the examination, because we will not respond to the licensing agency regarding your qualification requirements to sit for the examination. If any of you pursue this further, you will be dropped from the nursing program."

We were afraid and confused. We all assumed that she would be thrilled of our resolve to prove ourselves that we were nursing materials through one of the nursing licensing examinations. We did not know what to do. The following week, some of us who had not submitted the application for the examination, decided not to forgo the opportunity. We did not want to fail or to be thrown out of the registered nursing program by the nursing coordinator, since she had warned us. However, one of the students made a sensible remark regarding the practical nursing examination. None of us were on scholarship or government grants, but guaranteed student loan. The student said if we took the examination and passed it, we would get a job with it, and would be able to pay our student loan, but if we did not attempt the examination, and were failed or dropped out of the program, we could be in debt. He was not a pessimist. He did not mention anything about if we failed the examination. We all agreed and submitted our applications anyway. We all waited, and started studying for the practical nursing licensing examination. The school did not have a choice, but to submit all the required information and corroborated our claims that we were eligible to sit for the examination. We each received our admission ticket to the examination, which includes examinations date and locations.

We all stayed in our groups to study for the examination. The group discussion was stimulating, exciting and educational. It was better for us because we were relaxed, and were able to absorb information like a sponge in water. Things in the environment were utilized to explain nursing topics. Nursing textbooks came to life at the library and at student homes. This was andragogic learning styles at work, with student using life experiences to explain and understand nursing materials. We continue to study without any breaks, but to eat, use the toilet, exercise, and go to work.

The day before the examination, we all called each other at home. Those of us with employment, stayed at home. We all had an afternoon party. There were no alcohol, but juices, fried chicken and salad. We all left the party, which was at a friend mother's house at five in the evening. Many went to the cinema house to see a movie; others went home to do other things. We slept early, after we had all stayed on the telephone for five minutes to pray for help in remembering what we had learned regarding the examination. The following day, we got up early, and took the train to the examination location. We got there early and we began to talk and address some questions and answers in our practical nursing books. We each got to the exam hall, listened to the instructions and acted accordingly. We took the examination, and few weeks later, after painstakingly waiting in agony for the result, it arrived. It took many of us days to open the envelope containing the result. We were afraid of what the result might be. Many asked others such as friends or relatives or parents or their children to open the envelope with the instructions that they not be told the result if it was failed. Some even include a clause, some of which states, "Do not tell me the result if the letter states that I did not pass the examination." Others tried other methods of see and tell by their relative regarding the envelope containing the practical nursing examination result.

None of us were bold to tell each other if we passed or failed the practical examination for the whole months. We were all afraid of making our peers unhappy. We all kept the secret of our examination result to ourselves. A month later, after we had all got ten our result, the nursing coordinator arrived to give us her usual lectures. She was the one who let us know that we had all passed the practical nursing licensing examination. It was after that announcement that we all began to talk about what we had gone through opening and concealing the result of the examination.

The last semester was extremely hard for all of us. The materials discussed in class were not the material covered in our quizzes, tests and class exams. We knew that the nursing coordinators meant what she said about failing and dropping some students. Why now? We had all passed the practical nursing licensure examination. We had proved ourselves, both of whom English was their first language, and those of whom English was their second language. She had warned us and she was going to show us, who was the boss. Every student who had not been passing the quizzes, tests or class examinations were now passing with distinctions. The nursing coordinator was not happy. She accused one of the professors of giving students information about quizzes, tests, and class examinations. We all continued to do extremely well, however, before the final examination for graduation we were all called in to the nursing department office. One by one we were all interviewed by all the nursing instructors, with the nursing coordinator present, regarding the final examination. Many of us whom English was our second languages were told we needed miracle to pass the final examination. The miracle was that some had to get 96%, others 97%, and some 99% to pass the semester for graduation. We had been told we were on our way to graduation, but now, needed divine intervention to graduate. Those who were working among us quit their employment. We all moved from our rented homes with each other to simplify financial life to be able to afford the opportunity to study. We studied day and night using examination based question and answers textbooks for registered professional nursing.

The day of the final examination came, and we all arrived early as usual. We all sat in front of the school library, trying to get more information into our heads by reading our textbooks. The wishes of everyone was that the information in the textbook could get into their heads with little efforts. We have studied very hard for the examination. We had burnt our candles at both ends, and yet we still felt enough was not enough. We had covered two years of information through numerous nursing textbooks, which had taken probably five to ten years to write and published in two months.

The time was imminent, and some of us took the opportunity to visit the bathroom. Some were having loose stools due to the stress from the anxiety or fear of not knowing what to expect on the final exam. We had been warned, and threatened by the nursing coordinator, and she was in the mood to fail or drop some of the students. Our good result from the Licensed Practical Nursing Examination was not good enough for her to trust us that we would not let the college down on the Registered Professional Nursing Licensing Examination.

Our body began to go through changes due to the anxiety of the examination and many chemical hormones were being secreted. These changes resulted in diarrhea for some students and emesis for some students. It was what might be described as "fight or flight syndrome." It is our body's reaction to impending doom or harm, both perceived and not perceived. There was homeostatic imbalance as a response to the stress of the examination and the threat of the nursing coordinator. We experienced an increase in blood pressure, hormone, and psychosomatic symptom as soon as the time of the examination approached. If it was ideal or sensible to run away and not take the examination that day, many of us would have taken to flight. It was not an ideal situation to run because the examination was to determine our graduation. We all resolved to take the final examination no matter what the outcomes was going to be for us.

We entered the hall and took our sit. Majority sat in the back of the examination class for whatever reasons. We were told to leave our books outside the door, and we all did. No calculator, or wrist watch with calculator or any palm pilots were allowed in the examination class. The exams papers were given to us, and they were multiple choices as usual. The problem of the foreign students was that they were not familiar with taking multiple-choice exams. In many of the French and British colonies, the examinations are often in the form of essays. As a student, you are required to demonstrate your knowledge through explanation of the given topics or questions, to convince the examiners or the teachers that you understand what you had been taught in class. Multiple-choice questions often referred to as objective questions are rarely used in schools and national examinations. As such these students were not equipped to pick the best answers out of four or five choices in United States colleges and national multiple-choice questions. They now have to take classes or research ways to effectively pick the right answers in multiple-choice examinations. It was a dilemma, but not a difficult task. We all learn to dissect multiple-choice questions, as part of our nursing education.

We all took the final examination, and walked out of the examination class looking morose and melancholic. We were not sure or confident of how or what we did relative to the final examination. Every answer to each question was similar and had the same meaning, except in different words. We were expected to pick the best, and knowing the best in one hundred and fifty questions within one and half hours, was added pressure. In addition, we could not forget the threat of the nursing coordinator. We were under a lot of pressure to pass the examination as expected.

We wanted to graduate that year with our friends and group. We do not want to be left behind. We had become a family, that we could not imagine anything but moving forward together. Besides, many of us were up to our neck in expenses, that we do not see any other ways but to graduate that year with our peers.

After the previous semester, the nursing instructors and the nursing coordinator had begun to be fearful of the students they had deliberately failed or dropped out of the program. They could not go alone to their vehicle or attend school or come to class alone without escort. We even heard of situations in which students or school securities had to escort the instructors to the bathroom. Every evening, some of us who were men, were requested to escort the instructors to their vehicles. We did, but never knew why. Eventually, we figured out the reason the instructors needed escorts, the nursing instructors were paranoid. The nursing instructors had become victims of their own threats and errors in judgment by introducing fear tactics, and by provoking students. Students were provoked through exclusion from their dreams of becoming a nurse on the basis of their ethnic background and language. Students were provoked by verbal threats by instructors, of failure or expulsion or being told that they were not nursing materials.

Now that the tables have turned, the instructors began to fear reprisal from students that have been failed, despite giving the nursing program all their best. They gave the program all they have gotten and lost, not because they do not have what it takes to make it to graduation, but because they were judged by instructors, as unfit to be nurses or would not pass national examination on the first try. The instructors were also afraid, because they never knew the students. They had come to realize something that many governments and intellectuals knows, but never admit, that, "frustration breeds resentment and resentment breeds violence." Frustration often stems from lack of support either from government, society, friends and relatives. The frustration, if left unchecked, by accepting defeat and without taking your burden to God for help, could result in deep hatred (resentment). The resentment or deep hatred could result in violence if the initial problem responsible for the resentment persisted; and emotions are left unchecked and without any balance.

The students were nursing materials. They possessed all the qualities of nursing, love of people, and desire to help others. They desire to be nurses, so, as soon as they were failed or dropped from the program at our college, they transferred to another college to complete their nursing education. They returned to tell us about their wonderful experiences at their new colleges, and some of them became our colleagues at work, eventually.

A week after the final examination, all the other departments had released their result of the final examination, except our nursing department. On the day of the pinning ceremony, we were to report to the nursing department at nine in the morning. We were to be informed of our fate as to the graduation that year or not. Each of us was called in to the office of the nursing coordinator to listen to the instructors of what they think should be our end that semester.

It was a long day for many of us. We were all sad, and anxious. Each one of our peers, that entered the nursing coordinator offices left in a good mood. At one in the afternoon, we all heard the instructor's final words. They still insisted, they should have failed many more of us or that they should have dropped many of us. I do not know how many more they could have drooped. It was sixty students when we started; out of the sixty students, only nineteenth made it to graduation. How many more could have been dropped? Those nursing instructors just never quit. They were playing judge, jury and lawyer with our lives. They were convinced that they knew who should be a nurse and should not be a nurse. They did all they could to kill the dreams of many of becoming a nurse. I guess they rationalized their act as saving the world from impending problems of inept nurses. Ineptitude should not be a problem, in any society, if those who are empowered to teach do so as expected.

THE MYTHS ABOUT NURSES AND SOCIETY'S
PERCEPTIONS

Male nurses are homosexual, female nurses are prostitutes, and it is a taboo for male nurses to work in obstetrics or maternity wards, were common myths in most society, whether among the illiterate or the educated.

In Africa, male nurses are not seen as homosexual however, they are regarded by the health consumers as doctors or doctors in training. The reason is that nurses are generally female in many rural areas in Africa. When the villagers travelled to the city and see a man in white uniform, the assumption is that he must be a doctor. He would be called doctor until someone or he decided to correct the patient, and tell them his profession.

The African doctors also contribute to this ignorance that nursing is a female profession and that male nurses are doctors in training. In 1991, after ten years in United States, I travelled to Nigeria to see my mother. The trip was exhausting. I was physically drained. I had forgotten about the long hours on the plane, and the confusion and chaos of Nigerian airport in Lagos. After, I got home, I had a chest pain. My mother told me to go to the hospital. I went to the hospital and there was a male nurse at the General Hospital in Lagos, assisting the doctor in assessing each patient. His uniform was different. He had a white top and a white bottom pant. The doctor had on a lab coat. The patients were referring to the man in the white top and bottom clothes as the doctor, and the real doctor did not attempt to correct them. I asked why he did not help the patient understand the difference between the doctors and male nurses. His answer was, "why should I? They are content and satisfied with the care they are getting, and besides, it makes my life simple." I walked away after the doctor gave me my prescription for pain medication. I could not understand what he meant by "it makes my life simple." His life was already simple. He did not have to be concern about lawsuit from Nigerians. Malpractice insurance is not known or does not exist in Nigeria or most African countries. The doctors are not accountable to anyone. They just play doctors and act like gods. I finally concluded that he meant having little to do, since the male nurse his regarded as the doctor, and he was playing the part already.

Growing up in Nigeria, I often heard people call nurses prostitute. It is the same in other countries, the only difference is that the words are not as pronounced or loudly heard as it is in other parts of the world. There are two reasons the society may feel that nurses lack morals. One is ignorance of the demand of the profession, and the other is the nature of the profession and the fact that majority of the nurses are females.

As it is in many countries, nurses work in shift. The hospital or health care institution may have two or three shift, depending on its cost effectiveness. If it is two shift, it may be twelve hours day and twelve hours night, and if it is three shift, it would be three eight hours shift divided into day, evening and night shift. The nurses are rotated from shift to shift in Nigeria, and also in advanced countries like United States. A nurse may work day shift for some time and when it is her or his turn to rotate to evening or night, he or she would be rotated. The shift change may interfere with pattern of sleep. For example, a person who his or her body had been used to sleeping at seven at night may now have to readjust or find ways to sleep at eight in the morning. This is due to the fact that he or she has now been rotated to evening or night shift. The same scenarios will apply to those nurses who were on evening or night, but now have to be rotated to a new shift.

It takes a lot of time to get readjust to another time of sleep. This causes changes in hormonal balance, which could result in mood changes. The nurse may be cranky, sad, unhappy, or not in the mood to socialize after work, however these changes never affect quality of work. It may take some time to get adjusted to new hours of sleep. The demand of work may appear higher than the previous shift and at times it is. This may cause the nurse to stay after work beyond contracted time to complete his or her assignment. This happened almost every day. I could not remember a day of which I left work early or at the exact time I am supposed to close from work. It is always one to four hours after the expected time of closing. It is the same for all nurses. The perception of many, especially the ignorant boy friend, girlfriend, husband, and wife is that the nurse is having an affair. The husband may not ask his wife any questions or understand the cause of the changes, but assumed the worst and provoke his wife into a cause for physical abuse. The wife who is not a nurse may act in a different manner, but her action may result in verbal or physical abuse too.

For example, a nurse on the evening shift in a medical-surgical unit had five admissions. There were numerous problems relating to doctor's order and patient's family issues. The nurse had to attend to all the issues on the unit, and also complete the admission before she leaves for home. She had another nurse with her, but she was a Licensed Practical Nurse. She cannot do physical assessment according to policy and the state regulations.

The nurse called her husband at home that she would be home late as usual. The husband was not at home, but she left messages. The husband got home, and I presumed, he did what he often does when his wife was not at home. At four in the morning, the rattling of keys in the front door woke him up. He got up. He examined the clock on the wall as he had always. It was four in the morning. He was angry. He was fuming. He must have been like a bull ready to charge at a bullfighter.

"Do you know what time it is?"

"Yes. I know what time it is"

"You know what time it is? Are you crazy? Don't you have any shame coming home at this hour? Every respectable woman had been home since eleven last night. Why are you doing this to me? If you want to prostitute yourself, why did you marry me? Heh! When I proposed to you, why did you say yes?" According to my co-worker, her husband continued talking, analyzing, and second-guessing her until the morning. She did not have any sleep until her husband left for work. She loved her husband, and she did not want to do anything to break the marriage. The second day, she made all attempt to complete her work on time, but it was impossible. The drama continues, and her husband began to tell everyone about his wife. The ignorance of the profession and the demands of the job cause everyone closed to the couple to label the nurse as a prostitute. Her reason for coming late was attributed to sleeping with her doctors and co-workers. The recommendation by friends and in-laws to the husband was to divorce her.

In working with doctors and other nurses, it is possible to develop a closeness or bond of comfort in times of trouble. For example, nurses and doctors experiences bad situations everyday on the job. It may be the death of a patient in their care or a patient who was near death, but was saved. These and many other health emergencies like it tend to bring people together. This is because they understand one another in terms of the experiences, and thereby feel they are in the best position to comfort each other. This they often do aside, either by hugging with a shoulder to cry on. To the extent that these nurses and doctors look forward to the next time they would be working together. It is often a platonic friendship, and sometimes it is not. The relationships are healthy some of the times, but not healthy some of the times. Some found their future wives or husbands at their places of work, and why should nurses and doctors be different? This does not translate to the conclusion that nurses have uninhibited sexual drives or desires secondary to their profession.

The other reason nurses are called prostitutes is the nature of the profession, and the fact that the 97% of nurses are females. The perception is that, by nature, women are kind, considerate, and permissive. The belief of women permissiveness is global. It is almost inherent or embedded in human brains from birth. For example, a man may sleep with every woman in the neighborhood, and would never be called a prostitute. If possible, the society will even praise him or reward him for his action. In high school, boys make themselves look good by claiming to sleep with many girls in the school or in their neighborhood. If a woman or a girl should be seen coming out of another man's house or backyard, she would be labeled a prostitute. If she is found sleeping around, she would not only be labeled a prostitute, she would be beaten. If you ask a woman for help, she may be inclined to help, but a man may need to be persuaded to help. It is not a new thing to hear somebody criticize a man or boy for acting like a woman. This proves that there are qualities regarded by society as being female and as being male. The society regards nurturing and empathy as female qualities, and aggression, and domination as male qualities.

This is obvious in ways that man has dominated the planet for centuries to its injury. Women have been in the background tending to things that are pleasurable and comforting to the existence of man. This nurturing quality perceived only to be of woman, is one of the reason nurses are considered permissive or loose sexually. The fact is, women are not permissive or loose as perceive by the society. In my observation, as a male nurse, the men are more permissive, because the society accepts, allow, legalize and promote the behavior in men as normal.

The Working Experiences: The Everyday Nightmare

It was just seven in the morning. The previous shift was just exiting. We all gathered to get report from the nurse in charge about the drama that unfolded the day before on the unit. After, we each received our respective assignment, and we all left the desk to make rounds and to introduce ourselves to our patients.

The telephone rang. One of the nurses answered it. It was a spouse of a patient on the other side. She was yelling and screaming that the nurse holding the telephone could not bring the receiver closer to her ear. She did not allow the nurses to respond, she just continues to vent. After she had finished venting, she hung up the telephone. We went to the room to talk with the patient. He did not have any complain nor did he had any problem with the previous shift. We decided to call back his wife to find out what she was trying to tell us. She blamed us for not stopping her husband from waking her up at night. Apparently, the husband called her every night to complain or make inquiries about different things not relating to the hospitalization.

We provided a large print clock for the husband to be able to tell the time and made calls at appropriate time, and not when the wife was sleeping. We asked the patient if she would like something for sleep at night. He claimed he was not having trouble sleeping. He only missed his wife. The wife did not see it that way. She threatened to commit suicide if the husband would not stop calling her during the night. We refered the situation to the social worker and continued to care for the patient until discharge.

The wife visited everyday as if nothing had happened, but had other complains. She requested to review her husband medications. We had been informed by the husband to allow her to review them, and she was named as the health care proxy. She reviewed the ordered medications, and requested changes to be made to the medications without any reasons. The doctors were informed. The patient was consulted and he referred us back to his wife. Meetings were held to explain the significance of the medications and therapy to the desired patient's outcome. The wife explained that she had asked people and had gone online to examine the adverse effects of those medications and she thought they were not good for her husband. The medications were changed as requested, however the practice becomes everyday routine as soon as the wife came to visit. The time spent in the discussion could have been put to better use. There were those who felt that if she knows so much, how come she did not sign her husband out, and take her home to provide the needed care for her. The husband was asked, if he was ever abused by his wife, he became angry and defensive. He laughed, and replied, "No." Nothing we did for the patient was ever good or appropriate in the eyes of his wife.

We were frightened of this patient's wife, because when she arrived at the hospital she often had complaints. The complaints were often not medical but non-medical in nature. For example, one evening, she arrived in a bad mood as usual. She stormed into the room her husband was sharing with another patient. She stormed back out demanding to know why her husband's bedside table was near the other patient's table. We explained to her that her husband was playing cards with the other patient, and that was why the table was on the other patient's bedside. She warned us never to let it happened again. We wanted to tell her to explain what she just said to her husband, but it may start another war. She continues to questions the nurse's aide, who had her husband if she provides water for her husband, and if her husband ate all his meals. The nurse's aide responded, despite the fact that her husband was able to answer all her questions. She asked about the kind of program her husband had watch that day, and why the channel had not been changed. The nurse's aide responded that her husband controlled the television's remote, and the channel. It would not be polite to take the remote control from him or change the channel. She went on and on, in spite of the fact that she was well aware there were patients that needed our attention. We called the supervisor to come to the unit to assist us in answering this woman's questions, but she said she was busy, and that we should do everything not to anger her. We were on our best behaviors until the patient was discharged home. To our surprise, the patient and the wife sent a letter and fruit basket to thank us for our excellent care.

Like any other profession, where people of varied ethnic background are employed, nursing have its share of subtle racism. We live in it, and we do not speak about it or even mention it. It is bad that we do not speak about the racism or tribalism, which exists in nursing profession. Being quiet about the racism or tribalism in nursing makes it impossible to address or solve. The reasons for not talking about it are numerous. One of them is the fear of being called a snitch or a trouble maker. The victim of racism in nursing are nurses and often considered themselves member of the profession and do not want to be seen as an outsiders. They tolerate the racism and absorbed its effects on their lives and impact on career development.

For example, a male nurse was passed over for promotion numerous times. There was a director of nursing position opened on his unit. He was not asked if he was interested in the position. He was more than qualified for the position. The vice president of nursing employed another female for the position. The male nurse asked why he was not consulted or why the position was not posted on the bulletin board for the staff, where those with the qualification within the organization could apply for the position. The response of the vice president of nursing was that, the female nurse employed for the position had a certification in nursing rehabilitation. It was later found out that that was a lie, the female nurse employed as the director of nursing did not have any certification in nursing rehabilitation.

Another position opened in the staff development, and the male nurse expressed interest in the position. He wrote a letter to the director of human resources about his interest in the vacancy as the director of staff development. The response was that the position may not be filled. This was another lie. Later the position was given to another female nurse. The same thing continued to happen over and over until the male nurse decided to apply for a director of nursing position in another organization. The idea was to see if there was something wrong with him or the way he speaks that would made it impossible for anyone to give him the opportunity to utilize his advanced nursing educational knowledge. He took the position and he perform the duties of the director of nursing, staff development, infection control, and reimbursement. The staff were organized, and well equipped as he taught them about the regulations and ways of doing things the nursing practice ways. They passed the Department of Health survey without deficiencies for the first time. It was a joy that he did learn something and that there was nothing wrong with him, the previous employer under the direction of its vice president of nursing were just racist.

Life continues on the medical-surgical unit, but in several forms every day. A female patient was being care for by a black male nurse. He did not have to provide other nursing care, but administered medications by mouth, and intravenously. He was caring for the patient for about a week, without complain, until one evening when the daughter of the patient arrived. He demanded to see the nursing supervisor, after she learned who her mother's nurse was. She told the nursing supervisor, she did not want the black male nurse to care for her mother. The nursing supervisor asked her why, she just said she just do not want the nurse to care for her mother.

The black male nurse was asked if he knew why the patient's daughter felt that way about him, he did not have a clue. The mother was asked when the daughter left if the black male nurse had did something to warrant her daughter asking for another nurse. The patient replied, "I don't know. My daughter just told me she did not want the black male nurse giving me my medication." She was asked if the black male nurse had done anything specifically to her or to her daughter. She replied, "No! I have had him for a week. He is an excellent nurse, kind and empathetic, but my daughter, do not want him to give me my medication, and I must listen to her."

The request, after a week, and without any complain from the patient was a mystery to all of us, but it was not new to the black male nurse. He had experienced discrimination and racism in health care industry in many forms, and the request by the patient's daughter that he stopped providing care for her mother was just another everyday expectation. He did not know he was black until he got to the United States. He had always thought he was brown like chocolate. He had tried to understand and educate friends and acquaintances that there are differences between the color black and the color brown and between the color white and the color pink. As a foreigner and a nurse, he was unable to grasp the ideology between calling a person who is brown black and a person who is pink white. A white colored person is pale and a pink person has a good skin color as long as they are Caucasian or Mulato or Albino. This is true as part of patient assessment. The dictionary defines pale as colorless or whitish. On the other hand, white is described as holly, good, and better. To call someone black is to describe them as evil, violence, and bad. This was the reason the word black was coined for the African. Their color is not black, but brown, and white people are not white but pink.

Eventually, he came to realize the word black was used negatively to classified brown skin people, and to oppress those of different colors other than white. Black is used to depict bad things, including evil, and white is used to depict good things, including Godly things. In many early American movies, blacks were painted as inferior, bad and evil. It was not clear why; however it could have been fear or lack of understanding of the African Slaves or fear of repercussion of mistreatment, abuse, oppression, disenfranchised, and neglect of basic necessities of Africans by the majority of American white.

The black male nurse was assigned to another patient, and the other patient was assigned to another male nurse, who was white. The daughter came, she was not upset and she did not raise any issues regarding the white male nurse. The day the white male nurse was off, the patient was assigned to a black female nurse. The daughter came that afternoon, as usual. She was not happy. She had numerous complain regarding her mother's care. She asked if her mother received her pain medication, the nurse replied that it was ordered as needed, and that her mother often requested it when she was in pain. The mother was asked, but she replied that she did not want any pain medication, because she wanted to stay up to watch Oprah Winfrey on television. The daughter insisted that her mother took her pain medication. The nurse asked the mother if she was in pain and her replied was not now. The daughter went downstairs to complain about the black female nurse. Whatever she said was not communicated to the nurses on the unit, however, the black female nurse was removed from the patient assignment. The patient was provided a white female nurse.

When the black male nurse was caring for the patient, everyone thought he may have done something to the patient, and that was the reason the daughter did not want him to care for her mother anymore. Every eye was on him, scrutinizing and roving about him as if they were demanding an answer as to what he had done, which prompted the patient's daughter to request that he not be allowed to care for her mother. He felt rejected, and sad, and defensive, to prove his innocence that he was not guilty of any wrongdoing. One of the reasons was that, ever since that complain, the black male nurse had been on management video. He was watch like a hawk every day on the unit. He could not understand why no one believes him. He loved his job, and love people and does what he does for the glory of God, and not people. This way, he could never do anything bad to anyone. He could not harm any patient in anyway. Who would believe him? He is a male in a female dominated profession, and secondly, he is black. He did not have any ally, except the white male nurse, who also, did not get respect from the female nurses. He had life to live, he chose to stay on the unit and toughen it out.

When the daughter began to complain about the black female nurse, too, all the nurses finally realized that it was a black and white issue. The patient's daughter did not want any black nurse to provide care for her mother. She should have said that. It would have made life more bearable on the unit, because all her complaints and accusation got many nurses into some undeserved punishment.

It appears that as nurses, we are immune to abuse. It is not so. We are humans, but we are trained to evaluate every situation of things before we conclude or react. For instance, a patient is assessed in terms of psychological, physiological, environmental, sociological and spiritual problems before we formulate nursing diagnosis and goals. To help the patient achieve that goal or the desire outcome, we must come up with appropriate tools or interventions. The interventions has to be implemented, and eventually evaluated at the end of some specified time to see if it was effective in helping the patient achieve the desired goal.

In the process of doing our job, we get abused or hurt or harm by the patient physically, however, we are not to retaliate or defend ourselves in a way that could harm the patient. For instance, a patient requested salt and cup of soup for his lunch. The nurse reminded him that he was not supposed to have extra salt or the salty soup he requested. The patient got angry. "I am a grown man. I pay your salary by being here and if I want salt and salty soup, I should have it," said the patient. The nurse called the doctor. The doctor said, "Give him whatever he wanted. Just document the patient's non-compliance with medical treatment."

The nurse called the dietary department to request the salt and soup. The dietician reminded the nurse that the patient has congestive heart failure, hypertension, and he is currently on dialysis, and should not have the extra salt or the soup, as per his diet order. The nurse explained to the dietician that he had discussed this with the patient and his doctor. The dietician told the nurse to go and explain again to the patient the consequences of his choices of food. The nurse listened and entered the room to instruct the patient about the benefits of following medical regimen, and the disadvantages of non-compliance. The patient angrily asked, "Do you have my food?" He saw that the nurse did not have his request, he threw the water in the cup at him, and before the nurse could compose himself, he got up to strike the nurse. The nurse put up his hand to block the patient from getting closer to hitting him, and scream for help. Everyone came to help, but the patient was back on the chair. He was fuming with anger like he was ready to chop somebody's head off. He was calmed, and finally his salt and soup arrived. He ate and was discharge home the following day.

The third day, the patient died at home. It was said that the patient pacemaker was damaged when the nurse put up his hand to prevent himself from being hit by the patient.

The nurse was suspended indefinitely, pending the outcome of the investigation of the incident. Whatever happened to the nurse after, was unknown, however, everyone with the knowledge of what happened engineered some conclusion of the incident. Some claimed the nurse was arrested by the police, and was sent to jail. Other claimed he was fined and his license was revoked. Whatever the truth was, some undeserved punishment was meted out to this nurse for doing what he loved. Yes, it is true that there could be some physiological or psychological reasons the patient reacted the way he did. His aggression or combativeness on that day probably made it impossible to assess his physiological or psychological status before discharged home by the doctor.

Nurses are thought to be empathetic. Putting oneself in the shoe of the patient is something we have to develop if it was not part of a nurse's culture or home training. It is this empathy and love of patient, which often motivate a nurse to encourage a patient to participate in his or her care, or eat or comply with medical regimen. This encouragement can be construed as abuse or mistreatment if it seen as forcing a patient to do things he or she does not want to do. For instance, a patient lost interest in food. The nurse called the doctor to inform him about the poor appetite of the patient. The doctor ordered drug, which stimulate appetite for the patient. The nurse assesses the patient for other things such as effects of new medications, or psychological problems. Psychiatric consultation was ordered to rule out depression and other psychosis, which could have caused changes in appetite. Family was encouraged to bring food from home with the understanding that it must meet certain criteria relative to the patient's diagnosis for effective outcome.

It happened one lunch day, when a nurse put a spoon in the mouth of a resident with poor appetite. The family had been complaining that the patient was losing weight; and the staff new she had truly lost some weight, but they had to continue encouraging the patient to eat. They had conversation with the patient, and even try music or television with the food in front of her. With each encouragement, she turned her mouth to one side as the spoon advanced towards her mouth. The nurse continues to try until she got the chance to put the food in the patient's mouth, and that got her into trouble. The patient spit out the food at her, and knocked over the coffee, which burned the nurse on the chest and knee. She fell backward. She screamed from the pain of the coffee, but she was charged with the abuse of screaming at the patient. She was sent home for the day, and on returning to work, she was suspended for one week without pay. The hospital had adopted zero tolerance to patient abuse, neglect, and mistreatment. The zero tolerance was there, but it needed to be enforced without fear of union combatants. The only problem was in the case of this nurse, he was just trying to help the patient, but it backfired.

Sometimes, a clear explanation and verbalization of understanding could be a nightmare. A foreign patient with breast cancer that had metastasized to all organs was admitted to a medical-surgical unit. The patient situation, with radiation and chemotherapy was not getting better, but worse. A meeting was called to discuss with the family about the deteriorating health condition of their mother, sister, and grandmother. The family spoke English, wrote English, and understood English better than everyone in the room. The doctor began to explain the laboratory data, and the result of other pertinent test. The family began to cry. We consoled them, and the doctor continued with the social worker about advance directives and health care proxy, since the patient was now becoming confused and disoriented day by day. The patient was also present, as the discussion progresses. The family verbalized understanding of the advance directives, "DO NOT RESUSCITATE", but do not agreed with "DO NOT INTUBATE." They wanted to go home and discussed among themselves and come up with agreed answers

Two weeks later, they came with answers that we already know, from their body language and behaviors the weeks before. They chose to accept not to resuscitate their mother, but wanted her to be intubated if need be. It was confusing because in a cardiopulmonary arrest, how do you intubate without any cardiac interventions.

One afternoon the mother became unresponsive, she was intubated. The family was there. They insisted that everything should be done for their mother. A meeting was called again to explain "Do Not Resuscitate," and the family verbalized understanding and said they wanted it, because they understood that it would be futile to resuscitate their mother, sister, and grandmother. Hospice was further discussed with the family, and it was agreed that comfort measures was the necessary steps for the patient at this time. The family agreed.

One evening, the mother had a cardio-pulmonary arrest, and there was no pulse, blood pressure, and the only thing working was the mechanical ventilator. The doctor was called to come and assessed and pronounced. He came and he disconnected the ventilators, and pronounced the patient dead. He was walking out of the room to call the family, when they showed up on the unit. The doctor called them aside to give them the news, they insisted on going to the room first. The son walked into the room and he noticed that the ventilator has been disconnected, and that her mother color had changed, and that she was not breathing. He rushed to the nurse's station to tell us that her mother was still warm and that we should put her back on the ventilator. Every effort to explain to the son what had happened, only met with angry outburst. He became combative. He strike, and violently pushed one female nurse to the ground. The nurse did not call hospital security for help due to the loss of the family. They empathized with them and hope that they would understand they did not do anything wrong or insulted them in any shape or form.

The patient son began to hit and knock things on the unit to the floor. The hospital security was called, and they escorted him out and let the other members of the family grieved. The family threatened to wait outside for the nurses. They did and the police were called, but the nurses insisted that they should not be arrested. For several weeks, the nurses on the unit had to be cautious going home. Some of them found their vehicle tires slashed twice, and were reimbursed by the hospital management. It took months for the nurses to stop looking over their shoulders. The incident got calmed, but the scars on the nurse who was hit and thrown to the ground never gone away. She went on vacation for three weeks and finally decided to go into teaching. Her situation reflected a Nigerian proverb that states, "A person who defecate on the floor do not remember, but the person who clean it up never forget."

In some cases, the nurse never got out of the situation alive. In the case of a nurse in Africa, the confrontation between the family and the nurse was fatal for the nurse. As a matter of fact, this is every other day abuse by family of patients. They do not abuse the doctors, but the nurses who only follow the doctor's orders in providing care.

A patient with history of smoking for many years was brought in to the hospital. She was diagnosed with laryngeal cancer. The family was upset and un-consolable, as if it was the nurse who caused the cancer. The nurses were empathetic as usual, and continue to do so in-spite of the patient's verbal and psychological abuse. It was their job to keep calm and to care of the patient and family. The chemotherapy and the radiation took its toll on the weakened physiological system of the patient. The cancer was beginning to obstruct his airway, and he was immediately intubated.

The family was full of questions and the nurses were ready to provide answers, which they did with the doctor's assistance. They were concerned about how their father could develop cancer. People in their family had smoked cigarette for years and were never diagnosed with laryngeal cancer. The nurse questioned them on what age did the expired members in their family died, and if they were informed of how they died. They said some at the age of fifty and some at the age of sixty, but autopsy were never done or recommended. It meant the family did not know why those family members before their time died.

The nurse began to explain the research findings regarding the causative factors of cancer. Cigarette was implicated along with wooden stoves, and alcohol consumptions. The family could not understand why no one ever educated them about the danger of smoking and alcohol. They felt betrayed by the government, the politicians, and the corporate empire in the country. The advertisement of cigarette claimed that it is good, and African television role models are utilized to promote false benefits of smoking cigarette. The actors, actresses, and well liked famous individual smoked different brand of cigarette for monetary compensation for advertisement for the cigarette corporation. The people emulate this people and got addicted to smoking for life. In the villages, cigarette company claimed that smoking helps in driving away evil spirit. The people believed it and they began to smoke. They got addicted to smoking without any help to quit. Many had died of smoking without the understanding that the cause of death was the smoking. They blamed their neighbors, family, and other supposedly enemies their illness and death.

The family of the cancer patient understood that their father was not getting better as was explained, and as they have observed.

They came to the hospital everyday with their pastor, who prayed that God should not let the man died. This is another erroneous belief. God do not kill people. People kill people. It is the ignorance of some priest that God needs and angel in heaven and as a result takes someone's life. God as we understand him is love, kind, and caring. Nursing is a quality that could be attributed to God. He is not and cannot be responsible for anybody's death. They arrived with supposedly holly water for the man to drink. The nurses attempted to dissuade the family from giving the man well water or water from unclean sources, but the family got angry. The nurses continued to help, and continued to provide emotional support to the family.

Eventually the patient became diaphoretic, shivering and his body temperature rose; and continued to fluctuate between the administration of Panadol, and antibiotics. All interventions failed and the patient died. The family was upset, and went on a rampage, killed one of the nurses and injured many. The hospital called the police and the expired patient's family escaped. It was not a surprise that the family escaped, the police never showed up when their assistance is needed anyway. They often showed up when things have calmed down or after robbers have gone or there are no threats to them.

The hospital called the family of the nurse, and reported the bad news. The nurse's family was upset, and demanded justice, but from whom. The hospital staff and other well-wishers donated some money for the nurse's family. Scholarship fund was set up for the children's education. The news reporters were at the hospital interviewing people, and one of the people interviewed, have this to say regarding the murder of the nurse. "These kinds of things have been happening for many years. It happens because the people are suffering. They are jobless, and when the only bread winners they have died, they will take it out on the health care workers." Is it the health care workers that killed their breadwinners or the big multi-corporations? The big multi-corporations manufactures cigarette, and promote it as something desirable for consumptions. The nurses tried to teach people for years about the dangers of smoking, but the people just laughed. How is the nurse responsible for the patient's death? Why is it that the nurse is the one that get blamed when things goes wrong with the non-compliant patient? Why? The society just needed someone to pay for their loss, and the nurse was in vulnerable position, and became the fall guy or girl, so to speak.

One morning a skilled nursing facility became a nurse worst nightmare. The nurse was assigned to do treatment that morning. She entered the patient room and explained to the patient what she was going to do. The patient acknowledged understanding, but requested to be taken to the bathroom by the nurse. The nurse got the patient up and walked him to the bathroom.

In the bathroom, the patient closed the door. The nurse did not think anything strangely about the patient closing the door with her in the bathroom, because it was a big bathroom with self contained toilet with separate doors. The nurse told the patient to get into the toilet and do what he had to do. She was just about to walk out of the bathroom, to give the patient privacy, when she felt her clothes pulled at the back. The patient pinned her to the wall. Pulled up her dress, and opened up his pajamas, and let out his penis to rape the nurse. The nurse tried to scream for help, but he covered her mouth with his palm, and held her against the bathroom wall with his elbow. The nurse was struggling to free herself, but the patient was using the other hand to tear her panties to make way for his penis. The situation was ongoing for about five minutes when we finally heard the nurse screamed for help from the bathroom. We ran into the bathroom to see what was happening, and we saw the nurse pinned to the wall by this six foot tall patient in his pajamas. We pulled him from her, and we noticed that his penis was out of his pajamas, and there were some discharges from it. Some were noticed on the nurse's underwear and pantyhose. The nurse was in tears and shivering. Everyone tried not to ask questions. The patient was taken back to his room. The nurse was taken to the hospital by one of her co-workers, and from there was taken home. The doctor was called, and the family of the patient was called. Psychiatric evaluation was done and the outcome was favorable for the patient, but not for the nurse. She was out for six months. She was afraid and ashamed of what had happened to her. The nursing home used her vacation and sick days to pay her. When she ran out of available time, she resigned and went to work for another facility.

Once a nurse is always a nurse is what I was told. It is basically true. You are locked in for life. You could not see yourself doing anything else, but caring for strangers. Providing physiological, psychological, emotional, spiritual, and social needs for someone you do not know, and who could care less about your needs or your wants. Yes, this is the world of nursing, and it has its reward, not in financial terms, but self-satisfaction of seeing a sick patient smile, happy, and changed for the better. The self-satisfaction derived from nursing a patient back to health or self-care. It is a great joy to hear a patient say thank you for some or all your help, and even when they do not say it, it is enough to know that as a nurse, you do all that is humanly and medically possible for your patient, according to your institutional policy, and regulatory bodies.

A patient was admitted to a nursing home with physiological problem. The discharged information was vague. He appeared to have some psychological problem. He refused admission assessment, and all necessary nursing care. He had dinner that day because he arrived on the ward a little after six in the evening. The nurse's aide returned to the room to get the food tray, after the patient had completed his meal, he yelled at her and backed-up the behavior with a flung of water from his cup at the nurse's aide.

The offices had closed and the administrators had gone home, except the evening supervisor. The nurse went into the room to encourage the patient to allow the nurse's aide to give him a shower. He refused. He had a strong odor, which was overpowering. The patient in the other bed had begun to complain about the smell, which was making it impossible for others to breath. The nurse in charge called the supervisor to come and talk with the patient. She got up to the unit, and scolded the nurse to do something about the smell on the unit. The charge nurse explained that the smell was the reason she had summoned her to the unit. She walked into the room. She smiled at the resident, and called him by his name. She introduced herself, and extended a warm handshake to the patient. The patient took the hand and squeezed and squeezed and squeezed until the nursing supervisor began to scream for help. She tried to free her hand but she was unable to, because the patient was extremely powerful.

Everybody ran to the room to see the nursing supervisor in tears begging the patient to release his grip on her hand, but the patient was not moved. He had this flat affect like nothing was even happening. The facility security was called and they did all they could to free the nursing supervisor's hand. The doctor was called and the patient was to be seen by a psychiatrist immediately. The psychiatrist came, asked question from the staff and called the family to get pertinent information. The hospital, where the patient was discharged was called, and information about the patient was provided. He was combative during care routine, and he was non-compliant with medical regimen. He was on medical restraint at the hospital, which was discontinued prior to discharge.

The family refused to provide information, and all effort to get some answer to questions asked, from the patient, was fruitless. The psychiatrist finally arrived at a diagnosis, which every discipline had assumed to be the patient's problem, and he recommended some psychotic medication. The nurse was not happy. She had thought that the patient would be two-pieced and discharged to a psychiatric ward, but that did not happened. The administrator was called at home, and did not see why the patient should be discharged to the psychiatric ward. The nurse understood. It was a PRI period, and all the nursing home beds must be filled at all cost for huge reimbursement for care provided.

The patient refused the medications, and the doctor recommended that it be mixed in the drink for the patient. The nurses began to do that, and the patient began to respond appropriately to the staff. He became a model patient, until his other habit began to inflict punishment on him. He was a heavy smoker, and he also drank coffee. With nicotine, caffeine and diabetes, one of his diagnosis, it was just a matter of time before he was diagnosed with peripheral vascular disease.

He had a shoe, which he arrived on the ward with. The staff felt that the shoe was too tight for him, and got him another one. He refused to wear the new shoe, and the staff decided to remove the old shoe. The following morning, when the patient was being dressed, he asked for his old shoe. The nurse's aide replied that the old shoe had been thrown away. He got upset, and demanded in a loud voice that his shoe be found and brought back to him. The nurse's aide called the nurse to talk to him. The nurse entered the room, and the patient grabbed her by her breast with his two hands.

"Where are my shoes?"

The nurse was in serious pain. "Please you are hurting me. Release your grip on my breast and I'll find your shoes for you."

The patient did not respond. At this point, he was in another world. His anxiety had overpowered his sense of judgment or reasoning. The nurse screamed for help, when she could not bear the pain of the patient's grip on her breast anymore. Everybody who heard the nurse screamed for help hurried to the room. It took four able-bodied men to pry the patient's hand off the nurse's breast. She was in serious pain. Employee incident was filled out and she was sent home to see her doctor.

The patient's shoe was found and was returned to him. He continued to wear the shoe, but when his toes became red from the tight fitting shoes, they had to be cut in the back. The shoes were cut and they were not tight anymore.

The patient continued to abuse the nurses and was never sent to the psychiatric ward. Finally, he punched a patient on the nose. She was bleeding profusely. He was two-pieced and sent to a psychiatric hospital for evaluation. Other things followed such as reporting the incident. Investigation was done and the facility lost some money in one form or another. The man was later returned to the nursing home. They did not have a choice, but to accept him back. This is the world of nursing. We are here to care for everyone. We must find ways through the evidenced-based interventions to provide appropriate care for everyone regardless of their diagnosis. He had the same flat affect, and continued with his usual business of smoking and coffee drinking. He later hit another patient. 911 was called. The police came and the patient was two-pieced, and was discharged to a psychiatric hospital. He was admitted for four days and he was readmitted. On the day of admission, he assaulted a nurse, who went on disability for some weeks. The patient was still being care for, in spite of his abuses of the nurses. The nurses learned different approach, procedures, techniques, and all evidence-based clinical interventions there are to provide appropriate care for this patient. We are nurses, and our work is never completed, but continues like a revolving door, come rain, snow, or trouble on our unit.

Life as a nurse is interesting and exciting. Getting used to the daily changes in the way nurses are treated by patients demand courage and loving heart. The color of a nurse skin could make a difference in how his or her day would be. The problem is that patients or health care clients see black and white relative to nurse's skin color too. It does not matter how sick or ill some people are, they never stop being racist. For example, a black female nurse was assigned to a white patient. The patient regular nurse was white, and was off that particular Wednesday. The patient was very difficult. She would not accept any nursing care from the black female nurse. She came out in the hallway to verbalize her feelings. She stated in many "F" languages that she did not want the black female nurse, but her regular nurse.

She was informed that her regular nurse was off from work that day, and that the female nurse was the nurse covering for her. She said she would prefer another nurse. The nurse was asked to explain what she did to upset the patient. She replied that she had not done anything but introduced herself to the patient as was the custom. The patient was assigned to another black female nurse.

As soon as the patient saw her, she said, "What is this? African nation? Don't you people have other white nurses? I meant people of my color. This black nurse stink, and frankly speaking, all black stinks."

The black female nurse heard what the patient said, and she burst into tears. She was taken to the nursing office. She was consoled. The nurse did not stink nor have any body odor. It was established by everyone close to her, but to the patient, she stinks. The nurse went into the bathroom. She lifted up her hand above her head to smell her underarm. She did the same with all reachable parts of her body. She did not have any body odor. She asked other patients she had been working with that morning if she had an offensive odor, for the purpose of making bodily hygienic changes. They all responded that she did not stink.

One of her patient, who overheard the conversation in the hallway, explained to the nurse, what the patient who had called her human skunk meant. The patient explained that to be called a human skunk did not necessary meant that she had a body odor. She explained that it was a term used by many racists to insult those whom they considered inferior to them. The nurse finally understood the situation she was with the patient who had refused her care. The patient was assigned a white female nurse. She became satisfied and compliant.

THE PUSH FOR HUGE PROFIT, AND
INCREASING INTENSITY OF LABOR

Many health care facilities were once non-profit organizations. They did not make profit, and if they did, the profit was reinvested into the health care facility. The money was used for something new, repair existing structures, staff education, or other things to improve patient outcomes. Implementation of agreed or important research findings for the benefits of patient and staff was often achievable and quick. Going on vacation and taking personal days were done in an atmosphere of trust and in peace. Health care administrators gave bonus to deserving employees at the end of the year. Nurses were not just employees they were also the facility customers. Patients or clients were treated on arrival whether they have insurance or not, whether insurance was adequate or inadequate. There were no pretext nor lies not to treat.

Today, almost all health care industry is for profit. They even sell shares to the public and distribute dividends. The way the nurses work has changed. The way things were done changed. Materials used become scarce, and nurses have to improvise. The health care industry was revolutionized in a decade by the government and big corporations for push for huge profit.

It all started with the tightened control over Medicare, Medicaid, and other medical insurance. It used to be that the health care industry including private doctors and home care company could charge just about any amount for the care provided to individual patient. On any given day on American street, you could see people lined up on some street to see a doctor. Majority of these people do not have any health problems for which to consult the doctor. They are at the doctor's office to get a prescription for medications such as narcotics to use for psychological pain or to sell on the street. The doctor in turn would bill the Medicare or Medicaid or whatever medical insurance company was provided by the patient. The cost to the government would not be just about the prescription, since there must be health problem to prescribe pain medication or any medication. The doctor's office documentation would reflect presentation of health problems by the patient, for providing the patient with the prescriptions.

At the hospital, nursing homes, and other health related facilities, Medicare, Medicaid and other medical insurance were either assumed charged twice for services provided or assumed charged for services they did not provide. The cost to the government and private medical insurance company was becoming expensive and beyond expectations. It was assumed that it was obvious that many doctors and health care providers were taking advantage of the Medicare, Medicaid, and the private insurance system. Unnecessary procedures, test and other diagnostics tests were assumed being ordered or were assumed not ordered, but were charged to Medicare, Medicaid or private insurance company.

The situation could further be illustrated in a different way. For example, a father (the government or private medical insurance company), provided his children (the society) with money (Medicare, Medicaid, and other medical insurance) with which to care for self. The money was deposited in the bank. The father did not specify how much could be withdrawn at certain times or how could be spent on different items. Some of the children saw unlimited opportunity to enrich and change their lives for better or for worse. They decided to spend the money on what they want and not on what they actually needed. False claims were assumed made against the account and funds were collected. The father returned to see what had happened to the money and how some of the children had wasted the money, he decided to make certain changes.

In 1973 Congress passed the Health Maintenance Organization Act to curb unnecessary waste and abuse of Medicare, Medicaid, and other medical insurance, in the name of not-for-profit. This was the first managed care program implemented by the government of United States. Its intention on paper was to reduce unnecessary health care costs through a variety of mechanisms, including: economic incentives for physicians and patients. The Managed Care System control cost by dictating to the doctors, and health care industry what to do and what not to do for patient. Information about the patient's condition and reasons for tests and procedures are required for reimbursement. Incentives are provided to doctors or health care industries that follow the script of Managed Care Company.

Following Managed Care System, in early 1980s, Diagnostic Related Group System was introduced. DRGs have been used since 1983 to determine how much Medicare pays the hospital, since patients within each category are similar clinically and are expected to use the same level of hospital resources. The original objective of diagnosis related groupings (DRGs) was to develop a patient classification system that related types of patients treated to the resources they consumed. Healthcare industry has evolved and developed an increased demand for a patient classification system that can serve its original objective at a higher level of sophistication and precision. To meet those evolving needs, the objective of the DRG system had to expand in scope. Today, there are several different DRG systems that have been developed in the US. The Diagnostic Related Group System becomes another payment system for health care industry. Health care industries are being paid according to the diagnosis of the patient. Medicare, Medicaid, and other health insurance company afixed a payment to a diagnosis, and when a patient with that daignosis is admitted to a hospital, regardless of what it cost the hospital to provide medical care to that patient, the hospital will only be paid that amount. Let me make it clearer by illustration. For example, the government pays only $20 under the DRGs for the care of a patient with the diagnosis of Fever. The hospital admits the patient, and the cost to the hospital is $50 dollars. The government will only pay the hospital $20 dollars. This applies to every diagnosis under the DRGs classification system. Every diagnosis is afixed a flat fee that the medical insurance is willing to pay.

All these and many more regulations were tied to reimbursement to control waste and misuse of medical resources, however, cost and waste is not controlled, but quality care is prevented. How? The health care industry began to examine other ways to make money. Research studies were conducted, and findings were implemented to increase profit. Cheap products were substituted for quality products. Patients were discharged as soon as procedures were performed to provide rooms for new admission. Many nursing employees were laid off, and employers began to experiment with unlicensed employees to provide care to patients.

The results were increase in the intensity of labor. The ward, which may have required three nurses prior to Managed Care and the DRGs system now have one nurse to provide care to patients. The wards, which require two nurses, now have licensed practical nurse in charge to reduce the cost of paying a registered nurse. Work becomes harder and difficult and stressful. Many nurses resigned to find work in another health care setting, and many left nursing profession entirely. This create a nursing shortage, which soothe the health care administrators, because now, they could claim that there are nursing shortages, and that is why the ward is staffed the way it is.

Many nurses that love nursing and the people that they provide care to and could not envision doing anything other than nursing, stayed. The result are health problems from overwork and stress from the demand of the job. For example, health care industry open twenty-four hours and seven days a week. Nurses are required to be at work every day except when they are off. It was not expected of a nurse to get sick or to call in sick. Calling sick is frowned on and discouraged by health care nursing administrators. Several policies were written to discourage lateness and absenteeism related to illness. The nurses were always afraid to call sick when they are sick; so, they self-treat and come to work. The result is delayed health problem, which manifest itself as congestive heart failure, kidney failure, pulmonary embolism, cardiac diseases and sudden death. In one hospital in one year, ten nurses, including licensed practical nurses died of stress related illness.

No one especially the health care nursing administrators, sees those nurses death as stress related. Their deaths were attributed to other causes, however, the nurses and other disciplines who worked with them know that their deaths were stress related. The American Nurses Association fought for safety, and improvement for nurses in health care industry, but the American Medical Association in partnership with health care industry owners continues to block those improvements in congress. How? This is done through lobbying and monetary donations to members of congress to block beneficial legislation to nurses.

Many nurses tried to protect their license by protesting unsafe assignment, only to be disciplined or suspended under the pretext of other things. It becomes harder to fight for safety and improvement for nurses since the necessary changes are not passed into law.

THE SURVEY, THE POLICY AND THE POLITICS

The significance of nurses in the care of the patient is underplayed by the doctor, and other disciplines in health care industry. Nurses are belittled and their contribution is seen as not important to the patient outcome.

In every hospital, doctor's parking is available in abundance. The government even designated both side of the street adjacent to the hospital for parking for doctors. The hospital administrators and other department have designated parking inside the health care facility parking lot, except the nurses. It is either they have to park on the street, away from the hospital or have to pay for parking. If any nurse park in the doctor's parking on the street, he or she gets a fine or have his or her car towed away. If a nurse park in the hospital parking lot, a large self-adhesive sticker with information on the illegality of the parking is glued to the car window or the car is towed at the expense of the nurse. In spite of the lack of respect from the government and the hospital administrators, nurses still come to work every day.

One morning, a nurse arrived at work. She drove all over the street, but could not find any parking space. She drove to the hospital parking lot; she was prevented from parking there because it was exclusively reserved for the doctors. She saw that the designated street parking for the doctors was opened, and no doctor car was parked there that morning. She decided to park there until her lunch time, when she would move it to any available parking. She was hoping that the neighborhood inhabitants would have gone to work, and there would have been space for her car on the street away from the hospital.

She punched in and began to work that morning. There was one incident after another. First, a patient was in respiratory arrest, and she had to call a code. Cadiopulmonary resuscitation was started. All the expected team arrived on the unit to assist with the code blue. The patient was intubated and transferred to the emergency room, and from there to the intensive care unit. The nurse had to sit to write her note after things had calmed down. As soon as she sat down, she was called into the room of a patient, whose intravenous line was now infiltrated. She removed the heplock and had to start another one. As soon as she inserted the line, it was time to pass medication to the patient. She rolled her cart onto the highway of the unit where she worked that morning. The first patient she saw was missing two important medications. She ran back to the desk to call the pharmacy that she needed those medications for the patient. The pharmacy replied that the medications can only be ordered for seven days at a time and he was not dispensing those medications until he got a new order from the doctor.

The nurse called the doctor to request an order for those medications she had to give the patient. The doctor replied that he was busy at the moment and when he got to the unit he would write the order. The nurse asked if he would just give a telephone order, the doctor said, "No!" He hung up on the nurse. The nurse went to tell the patient that she was waiting for the doctor's order to get the medication from the pharmacy. The patient was not happy. She wanted the medication now, and she had grown accustom to receiving it at that time of the morning. You could even say that she viewed taking those medications as the pillar of her physical life. She called her husband and children to complain about not getting her medication on time. Now, everyone began to call the nurse's station for explanation.

The first telephone call came at ten that morning. She explained to the husband that she was waiting for the doctor to write the order. It took thirty minutes for her to be able to get away from the husband, who refused to stop talking. She went back to passing her medications; then, another call came from the daughter. She was polite, and answered the telephone again on the same subject. Four people called between ten and twelve noon of that day for the same thing. She spent one and half hour explaining to the patient's family that she was awaiting the doctor to write order for the medication.

By this time, she had forgotten about the car she parked at the doctor's parking space on the side of the hospital. The traffic police came, gave the vehicle a ticket at ten. Another one passed by thirty minutes after, gave the car another ticket. She got a total of five tickets for the same illegal parking, because she was only a nurse.

Finally the doctor arrived; the nurse got the order and hurried to the pharmacy to get the medication. She hurried to the room to give the patient her medication, but she now refused to take them. She replied that it was not too late for her to take the medication. The nurse tried to reason with her in every legal way. She mentioned the doctor who insisted on coming to write the order, and she also reminds her that according to regulations, she could give the medication one hour before or one hour after. The patient still refused. The family arrived. The patient told them she had not gotten her medication. They ran to the nurse's station to demand an answer as to why their mother, wife and grandmother had not received her medication. The nurse was busy explaining to the doctor about the laboratory result that arrived that morning. The family stood there. The nurse kindly asked them to excuse her for few minutes and she would come to the room to attend to their needs. She just needed to speak with the doctor for a moment before he left the unit. The family got into the elevator to find the hospital administrator. The nurse was reported of being rude and incompetent. She was called downstairs to the nursing office.

She did know what she had done, but from the tone of the voice of the person on the other end, she knew she was in trouble. She informed the licensed practical nurse and the nurse's aide that she was going downstairs to the nursing administration office. She gave them work to do. Initially, she had divided the unit into two. She gave half to the Licensed Practical Nurse and she took the other half. However, being the charge nurse, she was responsible for all the intravenous medications, assessments of new admission, transcriptions of doctor's order and many more. She gets paid for charge duties, but not enough for what she does on the unit.

It was forty beds unit, but every drama on the unit made it seems like it was two hundred beds unit. She took the elevator and pushed the button for lobby. The elevator begun to move slowly down to the lobby, then she heard the announcement CODE BLUE, and her unit was mentioned. She suddenly pressed the button for her unit, but the elevator only responds to one command at a time.

She stared at the elevator ceiling, and could not come up with an answer, but she knows her patient need her up on the unit, now. She became anxious and desperate, but locked in the elevator until it gets to the lobby. The elevator reached the lobby, and she dashed out to the exit door. She jumped on the stairs and began to climb as fast as she could until she got to her unit. She raced to the room to see the ventilator patient being ambued. She asked them to stop for a second. She checked the inner cannula. The patient had a mucus plug. She flunged the inner cannula into the garbage, and inserted a new one in the trachea, and ordered the other nurse to continue to ambue the patient. The pulse oxymeter was 76% at the time the code was called by the licensed practical nurse who found the patient turning purple when she walked into the room.

The nurse had informed the staff to make round every fifteen minutes on the unit and to pay particular attention to patient on ventilators. Her decision was a good one, because the patient with the mucus plug would have died of hypoxia, if she had not been noticed on time to correct the problem. Now, she had to decide whether to go back downstairs or not. She hoped that the nursing supervisor would come up to the unit with everyone to assist with the CODE, but she did not. She called the nursing office, but the supervisor was not near the telephone. She left a message that she would not be able to come, but would see her at the end of her shift. She sat down to write her note regarding the patient. The doctor sat next to her to argue why code blue was called. The nurse said she was not on the unit at the time, but she think it was appropriate because the nurse on the unit needed help with the ventilator patient that was turning blue (cyanotic).

The doctor began to lecture her about code blue and why it was necessary to assess the patient before calling the code. The nurse new that the doctor was not listening to her, and that it would take another hour, if she stayed at the desk with him. She asked the doctor if she wanted to use the chart to write notes or order. The doctor said, yes. She gave him the chart and left the desk to do her treatment for the day.

At this time, it was two in the afternoon. The nurse had one more hour to the end of her shift. She became hungry. She had not had breakfast or lunch. The unfolding drama on the unit had filled up her stomach. All the mechanism and the chemical reactions responsible for feeling of hunger had been suspended during those dramatic moments.

She looked up at the clock. She suddenly screamed, "Oh! My God." Everyone at the nurse's station stick out their heads, and the patient who could walk came out of the room to see what was amiss. They asked, a second after the nurse echoed those words, "What happened? Is everything fine?" The nurse replied, "I parked my car at the doctor's parking on the street this morning when I could not find any parking. I was to move the car before lunch, but now it is 2:00 pm." As soon as she completed those words, she raised to the stairs. She jumped on it and from the sound of her feet on the stairs, they could tell that she was not walking, but running or flying. One of the patient walked to the stairs door, and said to her, "Please, be careful going down the stairs." She heard, and responded, "Thank you."

She got to where she parked her car; the car had gone. It had been towed at or before two in the afternoon. She stood on the spot with both palms on her head. It was an African expression indicating hopelessness and doom. She relied on the car to get things done such as taking her children to school in the morning, coming to work, and doing other chores necessary for life. She could not understand how doctors have many empty parking spaces, and she could not park in any of them, as a nurse. She could not understand why her huge contribution to primary, secondary, and tertiary health was not valued or seen as important just like that of the doctor. She began to doubt her decision for becoming a nurse. She wanted to start self-examination, but she saw one of the evening nurses driving around looking for parking, she realized that she had to go back to complete her assignment for the day.

On the unit she became quiet, and the staff knew something had happened to her car. They did not ask. They just comforted her by touching her shoulder, and telling her not to worry. She just nodded. It was all she needed to faithfully complete her work for that day. She wrote her note and gave report to the evening nurse.

She left the unit for the nursing office to report about her car, and to see the nursing supervisor. She had already prepared a disciplinary form for her. She was going to give her a write-up, and not a warning, because she had failed to report to the nursing office, as she had demanded that mid-afternoon. The nurse scrambled all over the hospital in search of a union representative to accompany her to the nursing office to get the write-up. She found one in the intensive care unit, but she was busy. She told her to wait until she gets report. She called the nursing office to inform the supervisor, who responded that she would be going home in thirty minutes, and if the nurse did not get to her before she leaves, she should not come to work tomorrow. The nurse tried to laugh, but she could not, because she already knew she would not be coming to work tomorrow. She had to find out where her car had been towed, and how to get it back.

The union representatives completed her assignment on her unit, and she followed her to the nursing office. They got there and were ushered into the director of nursing office. The director of nursing was there with the supervisor, who was going to give the write-ups. The nurse sat down, and so was the union representative. They asked why the nurse was being given a write-up. The supervisor explained that the nurse was rude to a family member that morning by using a foul language, and by failing to medicate the patient in a timely manner. The nurse explained her side of the truth of what had actually happened, but the supervisor did not believed her. She told her she was getting the write up, and she would have to attend a customer service orientation the next day.

The nurse refused to sign the write-up, and the union representative signed and requested a copy for appeal of the write-up. The nurse decided to walk to the security desk to lodge complaint about the towing of her vehicle. She was told her vehicle was towed by the government and not the hospital, since it was the government who designated the street next to the hospital as doctor's parking only. She went to the administration building to find out why the nurses do not have a parking space, after all, there were more nurses working at the hospital than doctors and other disciplines combined. She was told that the doctors were with the hospital on a contractual basis, and they needed to make them happy. The nurse replied that the nurses were on contract with the hospital too. The vice president of the hospital management replied that there were differences between the two contracts. The nurse asked for explanations and the vice president replied that one was more important than the other.

The nurse could not believe her ears. She opened the door and walked out of the office to call the City Department of Traffic. She gave the person on the other end of the telephone the plate number of her car. The person confirmed that they have her car, and that she should come tomorrow with $500 dollars to get her car.

She got her bag, and walked to the train station to board it home. She stopped by the sign on the street. Examined it again, and could not believe that doctors have a street parking and nurses do not. No respect for nurses for all their hard work, but she was happy to be a nurse. She would not trade it for being a doctor.

The third day, she went to the hospital administration building to look for the president of the hospital. She got to her office and lodged a complaint about the lack of parking space for nurses. She emphasized the significance of nurses in every facility, and especially where she worked. She made them realized that if all the nurses left the building or resigned today, the whole facility would have to close down. In the process, whether they close or hired new nurses, they would still lose millions of dollars. She told them what happened to her at the hospital two days ago, and that doctors have ample parking space, and nurses do not have any parking space on the hospital complex.

The president of the hospital replied that the doctors were on contract and that was why they have ample parking. She also said that their services were important to the hospital; and that they did not want them to get frustrated and leave. The nurse could not believe her hears. She echoed what the president of the hospital just said for emphasis. It still did not sound right. She decided to tell other nurses about her experience and what she was told by the president of the hospital. The news began to float around the hospital. The president called administrative meeting, it was rumored, and a decision was reached to give part of the parking lot in the hospital complex to the nurses. It was not easy, but eventually the nurses got a parking space on the hospital complex.

It was unfortunate that a nurse had to go through that experience of having her vehicle towed on the hospital vicinity, while at work for changes to be implemented regarding parking space. It was unfortunate that hospital administrators did not see the value or significance or the importance of nursing to provide parking space for them. I guess putting profit above services is what hospital and nursing home administration is now about.

Health Insurance Portability and Accountability Act of 1996 regulate electronic transaction in the health industry. It protects information of patient in the health care industry. Individual health records are to be well protected, and consent to share or provide health information must be obtained from the patient before information could be shared with any third party. This act changes the way health care worker had been conducting businesses. It prevents casual delivery of information over the telephone, as a result it creates hostile working environment for nurses.

HIPAA law was not intended to create hostile working environment in the health care industry, however, this was what happen as soon as it was implemented. For instance, most information about patients that was often given over the telephone by nurses now becomes problematic. The telephone ranged. The nurse picked up the receiver, and answered. The caller asked questions about the patient in Room 204.

The nurse asked, "Who are you, and what is your name?"

The caller replied, "Am Ms. X, and the patient in Room 204 is my sister."

"Excuse me for a minute, I'll be right back let me check something out." The nurse examined the printed face sheet in the patient's chart to see if the caller was named as one of the health care proxy agent. The caller's name was there, but still she could not be sure she was talking to the same person. She became cautious and replied that the patient is fine. The caller wanted to know the diagnosis for admission. The nurse refused to give the information, and refer the caller to the patient. Ms. X got upset. She became angry with smoke coming out of her ears symbolically. She stated she had gotten better response from a two years old compare to the information she just received from the nurse. She began to yell, and calling the nurse all kinds of foul names in the book. The nurse was patient. She let her completed all her sentences, and she explained about HIPAA to Ms. X, who replied that she could not give a "F" about HIPAA laws. She demanded to speak to her immediate supervisor. The nurse transferred the caller to the nursing office to speak to the nursing supervisor.

Ms. X was unable to get in touch with the nursing supervisor, but she left several messages in derogatory terms on the answering machine. At 8:45 PM, Ms. X arrived on the unit. She asked the doctor at the desk who was the nurse in charge. At first the doctor did not know whether to answer or not because of the demanding and disrespectful tones of Ms. X. Ms. X must have noticed that she was being rude, that she decided to greet the person at the desk nicely, and asked again for the charge nurse. The doctor replied that she was at the end of the hallway passing medication. Ms. X left the nurse's station to look for the nurse, who at the time was in the room attempting to silence the intravenous machine. Ms. X began to look from room to room, without knocking before she entered. One of the patient asked who she was looking for, she replied, "the nurse." The patient told her that the nurse just left the room. She moved to the next room, where she found the nurse and began to ask if she was the person she had spoken to about the patient in Room 204. The nurse told her to wait for her outside. She became angry that she began to shout at the nurse in the room. The nurse walked out without silencing the intravenous machine, with the hope that Ms. X would follow her. Ms. X did, but did not stop shouting.

The nurse tried as much as she could to calm the visitor, but she was unsuccessful. She paged the supervisor. She responded, and the nurse informed her of what was happening on the unit. The supervisor replied that she should handle it. By this time, some of the patients had gotten upset, due to the yelling on the nursing unit by Ms. X. The nurse continued to reason with Ms. X, who at this time was trying to push her fingers into the nurse's eyes. The nurse could not stand the disruption on the ward by Ms. X anymore, she called the hospital security. They arrived on the unit and escorted Ms. X out, who at this time began to shout she had been unfairly treated by the hospital staff. She called her sister in Room 204, who was immobilized due to Multiple Sclerosis to inform her of how she had been treated by the hospital staff, and how they had refused to let her come to see her. The patient called on the intercom for the nurse. The nurse responded. The patient asked if all her sister had told her was true. The nurse explained the whole scenarios and how it has unfolded, and how her sister had behaved. The patient, who knew her sister believed the nurse. She requested that her sister be allowed to visit her. She was called that she may return to visit her sister, but she cannot harass the nurses, nor cause any disruptions on the ward. Ms. X came to visit, but she made the nurses her enemy due to HIPAA.

Another incident regarding HIPAA started the in similar way however, the caller was not a family member, but a friend of the patient. She could not get any information from the nurse. She got upset, and called the patient to complain about the nurse taking care of her. She said when she called the ward to speak to the nurse about her welfare, the nurse was unable to provide information, and was rude to her. The patient, who was able to walk, got out of bed to speak with the nurse. She got to the nurse's station symbolically foaming at the mouth.

"Where the 'F' is my nurse?"

The ward clerk replied that she had gone to lunch. She demanded to speak with the supervisor. The ward clerk asked why she wanted to see the nursing supervisor. She replied that it was none of her fucking business. She kept her mouth shot. She called the nursing supervisor, who came up without finishing her lunch to see the patient. The patient complained that the nurse had not given her, her pain medication. She said she had asked since 9:00AM. She said the nurse was incompetent, because she did not properly dressed her surgical wound. She said if she got infection, she would file a lawsuit against the nurse and the hospital.

The nurse was called on the overhead speaker to come to the unit. She had just sat down to eat her lunch when she had her name via the speakerphone. She covered the food and ran through the stairs to the second floor. She got to the ward to see the supervisor waiting for her. She looked around to see any sign of cardiac or respiratory emergency for her to have been called to the ward on her lunch break. She did not see any. She responded, "It had better be good to have to call me back to the unit on my lunch break." The nursing supervisor ushered the nurse into a room, and informed her of the accusation leveled by the patient against her.

She explained what had happened that morning, about the friend of the patient calling the unit for information about the patient, and how she had refused to give those kinds of information. She further explained that the friend had called and requested her call to be transferred to the patient's room. She spoke to her about the refusal of the nurse to provide her with information needed to file some pertinent papers for her. Regarding the pain medication and the surgical dressing, she said the patient had received the medication, and the surgical dressing done by the surgeon that morning. The patient insisted she did not receive the medication. One of the nurses and the patient's roommate corroborated the nurse's statement that the young patient had in fact received her pain medication, and that the surgical wound was dressed by the doctors. The nurse was to write a statement for the supervisor, and she did. The other nurses too wrote statements, and the nursing supervisor wrote a statement of what the young patient's roommate said. All the statements were attached to the patient's complaint and delivered to the appropriate department. The conclusion was that the nurse should not provide care for the patient anymore. The young patient was removed from the nurse assignment and was given to another nurse until the patient was discharged.

If there were no witnesses, the young patient would have gotten the nurse into serious trouble. The pain medication she claimed she did not received was narcotic. It had been removed from the narcotic cabinet that morning, and had been signed for. If this angry patient, who was young, alert and oriented to place, time and person had succeeded in her accusation, the nurse would have been suspended or probably terminated. The situation may even be reported to the Department of Health, which could result in suspension of her license. It took several months to years for many patients and relatives to fully understand and accept that HIPAA was not refusal by nurses to provide information about patients, but government regulations to protect the patient, and enforce privacy of information.

As the government health care finance organization and the private medical insurance company continues to make changes to reimbursement, the nurses employers continues to make changes to how, where and when nurses work. Many changes took effect gradually, due to reduction in reimbursement for services provided. It becomes nearly impossible for many health care organization to function. Eventually, many community medical centers had to close up services to the community.

Prior to reduction in reimbursement, there were services provided by nursing employer, which has direct bearing on patient's outcomes. Those services were continued education on critical thinking and practical application of research finding to effect improvement in patient's outcomes and length of stay. Many health care organizations required their nurses to have at least fifty continue education credits per year. The seminars were paid for, and the nurses were paid for those days they had to attend the seminars. There were educational days and maternity leaves for nurses. If a nurse was interested in attending a nursing seminar, all she needed to do was to fill out a request for payment for the program, and submit it to the appropriate department. She would be given the day off to attend the seminar, and the seminar would be paid for. The knowledge acquired through the seminar was always useful to the nurse and also to the employer. The nurse would learn new ways or acquired new information to better care for his or her patient. The patient was satisfied, and would tell his or her friend about the good care she received and the health care organization would gets more clients. The importance of continuing education to nurses and health care organization is well known to the extent that many health care organizations encouraged their nurses to further their education by offering to pay for it.

Today, due to reduction in health care finance, as a result of managed care system, diagnostic related group system, and other regulation tied to reimbursement, all the enjoyable benefits provided by nursing employers, have been taken away. It becomes difficult to get vacation as a nurse. It becomes difficult to attend seminars, and it becomes difficult to even go on maternity leaves, as a nurse.

For example, a nurse, who had been slaving for one skilled nursing facility for twenty years requested two weeks for vacation to prepare and attend her daughter's wedding. The vacation was denied by her employer; and she called her daughter to discuss postponing the wedding. The wedding was postponed as agreed for another three months. She submitted another request for vacation, and it was denied on the basis that there was no one to perform her services. She requested that a nurse should be assigned for her to train her to cover her on her absence. The employer replied that it was too expensive, because they have to pay her and also hired another nurse to perform her duties. The nurse could not believe she would not be attending her daughter's wedding. She ruminated on the matter, and she concluded she had to resign. She submitted her letter of resignation to her employer. The employer refused the letter of resignation, but agreed to give her one week to attend her daughter's wedding. She thought about it, and she could not understand she had to travel to china to attend her daughter's wedding for only one week. First, she had to pay $3,000 dollars for her trip, and second had to stay on the plane for more than eight hours. She told her employer, she needed two weeks for the wedding. This was a nurse who had never taken a vacation in five years. She had worked hard for the company for many years. She emphasized all the good she had done for the company and her patients. The employer insisted she could only have one week. The nurse resubmitted her resignation letter to her employer. As soon as she did, rumor heard it that she was terminated under the pretext of incompetency.

Just like this nurse, many nurses struggle for vacation every year, and it is a war between the nurses and their employers to get vacation for different problems or to relax. The same excuses given by the employers are we need to find someone to perform your duties or functions or it is based on seniority. If the nurse died today, it would not be impossible to find someone to replace him or her to perform his or her nursing duties. The employers even refused to pay for vacation sometimes until you provide plausible excuses for your vacation. For example, a nurse got some news from home in Africa, that her father was seriously ill. She contacted her employer and requested three weeks for vacation to go home to see her dying father. The employer refused. She decided to request a leave of absence. The employer refused to grant the leave of absence until she provided a proof of hospitalization of her father in Africa. She called her sister in her country to tell them what her employer was asking. They laughed, and asked her if she explained to her employer that they were poor and lived eighty miles from the hospital in the bush of unknown village. The nurse said she would tell her employer the fact. She returned to her employer and informed them that her father was not in a hospital, but at home in the village, where he was being cared for by the relatives, and the community herbalist. The employer accepted her letter and told her they would make a decision about whether to approve her leave of absence or not by the end of the day.

The nurse consulted another African in the nursing department to assist her in explaining how things work in Africa, especially the culture and health beliefs. The man went to see the director of nursing and the director of human resources to educate them about African culture and health beliefs. This was to enlighten them about why it may be impossible to get a doctor's note or hospital paper to prove that someone's father in African village was in a hospital. The employer agreed to grant the nurse the leave of absence to go to Africa to care for her ill father. The employer used her vacation time to pay her, but it took two months after she had returned, with some help, before she was paid.

Nurses work become overwhelming daily because other functions are being added daily to their difficult job. The paper work is much more than before due to numerous governmental regulations. It becomes impossible to complete any assignment within eight hours. Many health care organizations are now changing from eight hours to twelve hours a day schedule. Still it becomes impossible to get paid for overtime. For instance, a nurse worked four hours overtime on a chaotic day with several admissions. She signed the overtime book, and informed her supervisor to sign the book for her to be paid. The supervisor refused to sign, claiming that she should have completed her work within the time she had to work. She reminded her of the admissions and other things that took place that particular day. The supervisor still refused to sign because she had been warned by the director of nursing not to give overtime, and if she did, she may have to pay out of her pocket. The nurse involved the union, and the union made an appointment to speak with the director of nursing. The situation was dragged on for some time before the nurse was paid for the overtime.

The next time things get chaotic the nurse did what she could and left the ward. When she returned the following day, she was told to get a union representative because she was going to get a write-up for failure to complete her assignment the night before. She got a union representative and she was discipline for not completing her assignment. The information they were trying to impart was that, she would be paid for eight hour, however, she must complete her assignment as a nurse before she leave the unit, even if it took her twelve hours.

In the nursing world, the solution to correction is always punitive measures. Every time the nurse made a mistake, the first thing the nursing administrator can think of is disciplinary action. It does not matter whether the mistake had occurred as a result of inadequate staffing or burned-out or sensory overload or domestic problem. The nursing administrators do not ask questions or find out why problems occur, they only think about protecting themselves from legal liabilities.

For example, a nurse was assigned to fifty beds unit one Sunday. She was to administer medications, both oral and intravenous, to all these fifty patients. In addition, she was to care for their wounds, documented on some patients, supervised the units and assigned task to available staff.

The nurse thought of going home, but was told that she may lose her license if she does. It would be abandoning the patient. She loved her job and she loved her patient, but providing care to fifty patients alone could be harmful. The supervisor told her to do the best she could. She listened to her supervisor, who claimed she had tried to find another nurse to come in to work with her. She tried to do the best she could.

At eight in the morning, she was called by the nurse's aide that a resident was in respiratory distress. She assessed the resident, and determined that the resident should be sent to the hospital for evaluation. She called the doctor, administered oxygen through a non-re-breather mask, then, she called the patient's family to inform them of the changes in his health status and the transfer. The family could not agree among themselves, which hospital to send the patient. The nurse decided to hang up the telephone and called 911 to request an ambulance. The patient was taken to nearby hospital. The whole scenario took the nurse one hour and half before she could regroup herself.

At half past nine, she assisted in feeding some of the fifty residents, and ensured that every patient got breakfast. At ten, she wheeled her medication cart out into the hallway and began to pass out the morning medications. She was medicating the residents and dressing wounds in between. She completed morning medication administration at two in the afternoon, and she immediately turned the cart around to give the afternoon medication. She was on her toes all morning and afternoon. She did not have breakfast and lunch. She was hungry, but she rather completed her assignment for the day, before she sat down to eat or use the bathroom.

At half past three, she completed passing out medications and doing treatment. She sat down to write her notes, and the twenty-four hour report. She left the unit at five in the evening. The following day it was found out that she had forgotten to give a resident one tablet of Vitamin C. The nurse was written up, and suspended for two days. It was her third write-up for the year. All occurred as a result of inadequate staffing. She did all she was equipped to do. She had to work, even if the situation was not safe for her, because she loved her job, her patients, and had mortgage to pay.

We sieve through numerous complains every morning. We had several meetings to find solution to the patient's complaint. The cause of the complaint was obvious to the administrators and the nursing administration, but they prefer to ignore it. The owner made profit from downsizing of direct staffing. Administration staff increases for no reason. Majority of these people walk around doing nothing. They never answer patient's bell. They preferred to go and find the unit nurse or aide who may be busy with another resident a mile away to come and answer the call bell.

Every day, whether in the intensive care unit, emergency room, medical-surgical ward, oncology ward, adult acute care unit, pediatric acute care unit, rehabilitation unit, sub-acute, or nursing homes, a nurse is delaying his or her urination or bowel movement for patient care. It is an everyday occurrence in every nursing unit or ward. The nurse have the urge to urinate or defecate, and something happened with the patient, the nurse had to ensure that the patient is safe, comfortable and satisfied before he or she can go to the bathroom. For many nurses, it has become everyday occurrence that their body has now become accustomed to delaying urine for four to six hours, since this is how long it takes often for the nurses to held their urine or the urge to defecate during patient care. Most of the patients are like children without any compassion, but desire to have their need satisfied, and the nurses ensure that the patient are happy before they satisfied their needs. The result is that the nurses occasionally become the patient, get sick and had to see their doctors. The irony is that many nurses self-treat and back to work to assist their patient with activities of daily living or whatever to ensure effective outcome.

Conclusion

These and many more are the experiences of many nurses daily on the hospital, clinic, nursing homes, adult day care, and other health care institutions. The experiences described in this letter are just few of what nurses encounter daily. There are good and wonderful things, which I could have added however, I want you to know that nursing profession is not as simple as reciting the alphabet. I do not want to tell you what you should do with your life or that you should become a nurse. I want you to make up your mind without any persuasion that nursing is your calling.

I am a nurse, and I could not see myself doing anything else. I love people, and I enjoy caring for the ill, the sick and even those who are healthy. The life that I have saved as a result of being a registered nurse had not only been that of the strangers, but also those of my family. It is a wonderful profession with many rewards in kind and not in cash. It is a selfless profession in which you give all of yourself for less in cash, but you are always happy.

Nurses have saved the life of policemen, firemen, politicians, doctors, other nurses, and every other people in every discipline you could imagine. Nurses are the everyday heroes that do not get respect from their government, employers, and neighbors. Every time a nurse makes a mistake, no one asked why the mistake occur or thoroughly investigate the mistake to see or learn why or how or when things happened. The nurse is immediately crucified by the media, the society, and the government. Everyone is ready with tires, kerosene, stones, and gasoline to lynch the nurse. The employer will make up files and punishment to try to paint the nurse as incompetent to deflect the liability or heap the blame on the nurse. The patient and the family would began to think of lawsuit and not to educate or instruct but to get rich as if that is the solution. The government, under the direction of a zealous prosecutor, who at this time is looking for opportunity to grow wings, would try every ways and tactics to make the nurse appeared heartless and worst than a murderer. Nurses do not get any respect or compassion or consideration or any help from any arms of the government. We are always under the microscope of everyone, and yet we still give our very best every day, because our love of people is unconditionally genuine.

I will let you think about what I have told you and what you have just read about the nursing profession for some time. I know you will make the right decision by making the profession of nursing your own. If you need any further assistance, please, do not hesitate to ask any registered nurse in your local hospital or call your State board of nursing. Thank you

Sincerely,
Your Loving Brother in the Profession of Nursing.

www.ingramcontent.com/pod-product-compliance
Lightning Source LLC
Chambersburg PA
CBHW021231280526
45784CB00005B/2060